Patient Safety and Quality Improvement in Anesthesiology and Perioperative Medicine

Patient Safety and Quality Improvement in Anesthesiology and Perioperative Medicine

Edited by

Sally E. Rampersad
University of Washington School of Medicine and Seattle Children's Hospital

Cindy B. Katz
Seattle Children's Hospital

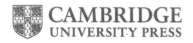

Shaftesbury Road, Cambridge CB2 8EA, United Kingdom

One Liberty Plaza, 20th Floor, New York, NY 10006, USA

477 Williamstown Road, Port Melbourne, VIC 3207, Australia

314–321, 3rd Floor, Plot 3, Splendor Forum, Jasola District Centre, New Delhi – 110025, India

103 Penang Road, #05–06/07, Visioncrest Commercial, Singapore 238467

Cambridge University Press is part of Cambridge University Press & Assessment, a department of the University of Cambridge.

We share the University's mission to contribute to society through the pursuit of education, learning and research at the highest international levels of excellence.

www.cambridge.org
Information on this title: www.cambridge.org/9781316642306
DOI: 10.1017/9781108125758

First published 2023

Printed in the United Kingdom by TJ Books Limited, Padstow Cornwall

A catalogue record for this publication is available from the British Library.

Library of Congress Cataloging-in-Publication Data
Names: Rampersad, Sally E., editor. | Katz, Cindy (Cindy B.), editor.
Title: Patient safety and quality improvement in anesthesiology and perioperative medicine / edited by Sally E. Rampersad, Cindy Katz.
Description: Cambridge, United Kingdom ; New York, NY : Cambridge University Press, 2022. | Includes bibliographical references and index.
Identifiers: LCCN 2022026022 | ISBN 9781316642306 (paperback) | ISBN 9781108125758 (ebook)
Subjects: MESH: Patient Safety | Perioperative Care | Anesthesia | Quality Improvement
Classification: LCC RD81 | NLM WX 185 | DDC 617.9/6–dc23/eng/20220801
LC record available at https://lccn.loc.gov/2022026022

ISBN 978-1-316-64230-6 Paperback

Contents

Section 5–People, Behavior, and Communication

A color plate section will be found between pages 82 and 83.

Figures

Tables

Contributors

David Buck
Associate Professor Clinical Anesthesia
and Pediatrics, Cincinnati Children's
Hospital

Rebecca Claure
Medical Director, Perioperative Services,
Lucile Packard Children's Hospital;
Clinical Professor of Anesthesia, Stanford
University School of Medicine

Aaron C. Dipzinski
Director of Ambulatory Services,
Ambulatory Growth, PeaceHealth

Nathaniel Greene
Congenital Cardiac and Pediatric
Anesthesiologist, Randall Children's
Hospital; Staff Anesthesiologist, Legacy
Emanuel Hospital; Shareholder Physician,
Oregon Anesthesiology Group

Eliot Grigg
Associate Professor, University of
Washington Department of Anesthesiology
and Pain Medicine, Division of Pediatric
Anesthesiology, Seattle Children's Hospital

Manon Haché
Associate Professor of Anesthesiology
at Columbia University Irving Medical
Center, Division of Pediatric Anesthesia

Cindy B. Katz
Manager, Surgical Quality Programs,
Seattle Children's Hospital

Daniel K. W. Low
Associate Professor, University
of Washington, Department of
Anesthesiology and Pain Medicine,
Division of Pediatric Anesthesiology,
Seattle Children's Hospital

Lizabeth D. Martin
Associate Professor, University of
Washington Department of Anesthesiology
and Pain Medicine, Division of Pediatric
Anesthesiology, Seattle Children's Hospital

Lynn D. Martin
Medical Director, Bellevue Surgery Center,
Seattle Children's Hospital; Professor
of Anesthesiology and Pain Medicine,
Adjunct Professor of Pediatrics, University
of Washington School of Medicine

Julianne Mendoza
Clinical Associate Professor, Director,
Pediatric Anesthesia for Liver
Transplantation; Co-Chair, Pediatric
Anesthesiology Professional Practice
Evaluation Committee, Department of
Anesthesiology, Stanford University
School of Medicine

Wendy E. Murchie
Pediatric Nurse Practitioner, Blood and
Marrow Transplant, Fred Hutchinson
Cancer Research Center

Sally E. Rampersad
Professor, University of Washington
Department of Anesthesiology and
Pain Medicine, Division of Pediatric
Anesthesiology, Seattle Children's
Hospital

Joan S. Roberts
Professor, Division of Pediatric Critical
Care Medicine, University of Washington,
Seattle Children's Hospital

Axel Roesler
Professor, Interaction Design, Division
of Design, School of Art + Art History +
Design, University of Washington

Douglas R. Thompson
Associate Professor, Washington
University in St. Louis School of Medicine

Imelda M. Tjia
Anesthesiologist, Texas Children's
Hospital; Associate Professor of
Anesthesiology, Baylor College of
Medicine

Kristina A. Toncray
Medical Director, Patient Safety, Seattle
Children's Hospital; Clinical Associate
Professor of Pediatrics, Associate Vice
Chair for Quality and Safety, Department
of Pediatrics, University of Washington
School of Medicine

Acknowledgments

We would like to thank Amy Pottharst for her meticulous work editing and proofreading, and our families for their unwavering support.

Introduction
Why Another Book about Patient Safety?

Sally E. Rampersad

Why another patient safety book? In the following chapters, you will be guided through not only the theory but also the practical application of tools that can be used to enhance quality and safety in medicine. Many, but by no means all, of the examples are drawn from the perioperative environment. Several of the lessons were initially used in other "high-reliability" industries such as aviation, nuclear power, and petroleum industries. We will include principles taken from these industries' safety cultures. These principles include:

1. Preoccupation with failure
2. Reluctance to simplify
3. Sensitivity to operations
4. Commitment to resilience
5. Deference to expertise

"Preoccupation with failure" refers to the idea that any lapse, no matter how small, could be a symptom of a system problem and should be followed up and resolved. Several small lapses could add up to a potentially severe consequence and must be addressed. "Reluctance to simplify" means that an organization takes time to understand the complete situation with all of the details considered and with varied opinions being valued and weighed rather than relying upon a "we've always done it this way" mentality. "Sensitivity to operations" is attending to the details of how frontline workers do their jobs and really knowing and understanding in order to have situational awareness. "Commitment to resilience" refers to the ability of an organization to be dynamic, to cope with errors that arise, to mitigate them and to be able to move on and to keep functioning. Finally, "deference to expertise" occurs when people are relied upon to do the jobs that they do best, without regard for hierarchy. Decisions are made by frontline people who have the most knowledge of the particular situation.[1]

In Section 1, we look at planning and preparation through the use of simulation and through the deliberate design of the work environment. The reader will see that through design, the right thing to do can become the easy thing to do. Through simulation, practicing the desired responses to emergency situations can prepare healthcare providers to better navigate emergencies when they arise, with no risk to patients.

Section 2 describes several Quality Improvement (QI) tools such as daily management systems, Lean, the Model for Improvement, and cause analysis. These tools can be used both to plan for QI projects and to analyze an adverse event after it has occurred.

Next, in Section 3, we look at ways that adverse events are reported and what can be learned from this reporting, including a look at national databases and pooled data sources.

Putting the tools into practice, Section 4 examines some projects undertaken at the authors' institutions.

In Section 5, we acknowledge that people are what make or break any QI efforts. There is examination of some of the "softer" patient safety skills such as effective communication. Stylized forms of communication such as handoff tools are described in detail, as are specific tools used to communicate and escalate a concern. Finally, we look at behavior and what it takes to change behavior to create a safer environment for our patients, families, and staff.

Since the authors started writing their chapters, the world has been gripped by COVID-19, a public health crisis unlike anything we have seen in our lifetimes. There have been many instances when hospitals have turned to some of the very tools described in this book to face this challenge. Simulations have been done to practice for the intubation of a patient with unknown COVID-19 status or known positive COVID-19 status.[2] Teams have considered the effects that COVID-19 will have on patients presenting for other conditions, such as labor and delivery. In addition, they have had to consider how to continue with proficiency training while maintaining social distancing and adequate protection for trainers and learners.[3] Lean methodology has been used to address the supply chain for vital testing kits and personal protective equipment[4] because worldwide shortages have threatened to undermine our ability to deliver care safely. In a very fast-changing world, I hope that you will find tools and ideas within these pages that will help you and your hospital to stay one step ahead and stay safe.

References

1. Weick KE and Sutcliffe KM. *Managing the Unexpected*. 2nd ed., Hoboken, NJ, Jossey-Bass, 2007.

2. Daly Guris RJ, Doshi A, Boyer DL, et al. Just-in-time simulation to guide workflow design for coronavirus disease 2019 difficult airway management. *Pediatric Critical Care Medicine*. 2020;21(8):e485–e490. doi:10.1097/PCC.0000000000002435, 10.1097/PCC.0000000000002435.

3. Kiely DJ, Posner GD, and Sansregret A. Health care team training and imulation-based education in obstetrics during the COVID-19 pandemic. *Journal of Obstetrics and Gynaecology Canada*. 2020;42(8):1017–1020. doi:10.1016/j.jogc.2020.05.007, 10.1016/j.jogc.2020.05.007.

4. Sheehan JR, Lyons B, and Holt F. The use of Lean methodology to reduce personal protective equipment wastage in children undergoing congenital cardiac surgery, during the COVID-19 pandemic. *Paediatric Anaesthesia*. 2021;31(2):213–220. doi:10.1111/pan.14102. Epub 2020 Dec 20. PMID: 33345391.

Use of Simulation and Patient Safety

Douglas R. Thompson

Introduction

Simulation has a long history of use in medicine; in fact, simulation courses on midwifery were offered in London in the 1700s using a "machine" to simulate labor and delivery.[1] Then, as now, simulation facilitated the acquisition of new skills and knowledge. Its use has the advantage of allowing realistic training without "practicing" on patients and the incumbent risk that may portend. The potential benefits of simulation in medical education seem obvious, and its utility has been well supported in scientific literature. Simulation has been shown to improve teamwork and communication,[2] and the use of simulation improves patient outcomes with decreased morbidity and mortality.[3] Although a broad topic, this chapter will focus on the use of simulation as a mechanism to improve patient safety and outcomes via identification of latent safety threats (LSTs), task training, and advancing team performance.

Simulation as a Means to Identify Latent Safety Threats

In healthcare, as in other high-risk industries such as commercial aviation or the nuclear power industry, the factors that predispose an adverse event may not always be apparent and may not be due to a singular error. A systems-based approach to improving patient safety in the healthcare system takes the focus away from blaming a particular individual or individuals for an error and shifts the emphasis to organizational or environmental factors that created the circumstances for the error to occur. Organizational factors have been referred to as latent risk factors or latent safety errors or threats. In medicine, this has been further defined as "system based threats to patient safety that can materialize at any time."[4] Simulation has found widespread application in the identification of potential LSTs, including equipment, medications, resources, personnel, technical skills, and knowledge gaps. By identifying potential LSTs through simulation, new processes can be tested before interfacing with actual patients.

Riley et al.[5] simulated obstetric emergencies with multidisciplinary teams of physicians, nurses, and support staff at six different hospitals conducting 46 trials over the span of two years. The authors developed their scenarios on the basis of actual sentinel events, and all simulations were video-recorded, allowing for the assessment of the institutional systems in place and the performance of the personnel involved. Following the simulation event, a facilitated debriefing session was held during which participants identified system processes that did not perform to the fullest extent and might contribute to an adverse event and poor patient outcome. The authors were able to identify 461 LSTs which were then subdivided into three broad categories: policy (procedures not being followed due to

3

Table 2.1 Improvements made by the neonatal ICU (NICU) leadership as a result of threats identified in simulation

Changes made within the NICU
- Calculators added to code cart.
- Adenosine added to medication dispensing system.
- Nursing education competency created and executed for adenosine delivery.
- IO infusion drill system education added to NICU fellow and APN skills lab.
- Nursing education competency created for location of defibrillator in NICU.
- Banding gun added to thoracostomy tube tote.
- Education competency created for use of banding gun and ties to secure thoracostomy tube.
- Protocol developed and education delivered on testing of defibrillator.
- Education competency developed on proper setup for storage of defibrillator.
- Defibrillator resource cards added to unit defibrillator.
- Revised angiocaths for premade needle aspiration kit.
- Malfunctioning electrical outlet in patient room repaired.

Changes made to the delivery room process
- End-tidal carbon dioxide detector added to delivery cart.
- Transilluminator added to delivery cart.
- Backboard added to delivery cart.
- Slide presentation developed for real-time use before congenital diaphragmatic hernia deliveries.
- Code (recording) sheet created and added to delivery cart for documentation of care.
- Additional RN now attends deliveries.

Change made within the hospital
- Hospital CPR Committee revised labeling for IO access supplies in code carts.

*IO, intraosseous; APN, advanced practice nurse; CPR, cardiopulmonary resuscitation.
Reprinted from Wetzel EA, Land TR, Pendergrass TL, et al. Identification of latent safety threats using high-fidelity simulation-based training with multidisciplinary neonatology teams. *Jt Comm J Qual Patient Saf.* 2013; 39(6): 268–273. Copyright 2013, with permission from Elsevier.

a lack of knowledge, skills, or training), with specific examples including failure to place an ID band on the patient and respondents not knowing their role in an infant code; equipment (unavailability of necessary equipment), an example being the absence of an infant isolette in the operating room for use in the resuscitation; and processes (system process failures), such as an inadequate blood ordering process in an emergency.

An important conclusion reached by the study authors was that many of the LSTs would not have been recognized if they had not been "discovered" or specifically called out by the participants during the simulations. It should be emphasized that these threats were identified without ever endangering actual patients. Endeavors such as those described in the study allow for proactive measures to be taken, such as additional training, policy clarification, system process improvements, or equipment procurement *before* an adverse or suboptimal patient outcome results. Undertaking this simulation curriculum is no small task. It involves huge resources, personnel power, time, and expense; these considerations must be balanced with the benefits of improved patient care. These considerations also speak to the importance of justifying the use of simulation.

In work done by Wetzel et al.,[6] the authors describe using both in situ and laboratory simulation in a multidisciplinary team-based approach with the aim of identifying LSTs to patient care. Similar to the work done by Riley et al.,[5] numerous LSTs were discovered in the structured debriefings and were categorized under equipment, medications, personnel, resources, or skill with 29 LSTs being identified during the in situ sessions. Of note, 22 of the LSTs were novel threats that had not previously been reported during the laboratory simulation sessions. This demonstrates the added benefit of in situ simulation. As a direct result of the simulations and identification of LSTs in this study, hospital leadership was able to target specific, concrete improvements (Table 2.1). As the authors conclude, "the subsequent clinical improvements made to the actual clinical care environment are the best objective evidence of the benefits of simulation."

Task Training: Deliberate Practice Makes Perfect

The traditional apprenticeship model in medicine wherein junior residents are supervised performing procedures by more senior practitioners is associated with inherent variability and leaves the trainee feeling uncomfortable.[7] Simulation training may offer a better alternative. Mannequin-based (also referred to as task trainer) simulation allows for realistic training in complex and potentially harmful medical procedures without having to put patients at risk. As such, simulation has found wide applicability in medicine, including disciplines such as obstetrics and gynecology, surgery, anesthesiology, and critical care. Furthermore, there is a robust body of literature that shows that such training improves success rates and, in many studies, improves clinical outcomes.

In obstetrics, shoulder dystocia may complicate 2% of vaginal deliveries. Despite the low incidence, shoulder dystocia may lead to profound and long-lasting complications such as brachial plexus injury, clavicle fracture, or even hypoxic brain injury, making preparation for this eventuality of paramount importance. To investigate the impact of training for this scenario on a task trainer, Deering et al.[8] randomly assigned participating obstetrics/gynecology residents to one of two groups: the control group or the group training using an obstetric birthing simulator. Subsequently, the residents were tested with a standardized shoulder dystocia scenario. The authors found that the simulation-trained residents scored significantly better in all evaluated categories, including the time to delivery. Importantly, although the number of corrective maneuvers that the trained and untrained residents could *describe* during testing to treat the shoulder dystocia did not differ, the trained residents were more likely to *perform* "critical" initial maneuvers. The authors suggest that this difference "demonstrates that the practical application of this 'book knowledge' can be significantly enhanced by simulation training." This study suggests that prior simulation training may improve outcomes in patients with shoulder dystocia.

A subsequent study provided further and stronger evidence of the utility of simulation training and improved outcomes in treating shoulder dystocia in the delivery room. Draycott et al.,[9] in a retrospective analysis, compared management and neonatal injury associated with shoulder dystocia before and after simulation training, which included the use of a shoulder dystocia task trainer (Figure 2.1). After introducing the training, clinical management improved (significantly more maneuvers for the resolution of shoulder dystocia used) and neonatal outcomes also improved. The authors found a statistically significant reduction in neonatal injury and neonates with a brachial plexus injury at birth.

Central line insertion is a commonly performed procedure in many hospitals, often done in the sickest of patients who can ill afford a procedural complication. Given the high frequency with which this procedure is done, several studies have examined the impact of task trainers. Evans et al.,[10] in a prospective, randomized, controlled study of first- and second-year residents, measured success rates for first cannulation and central venous catheter (CVC) insertion on hospital patients. The intervention group of residents underwent

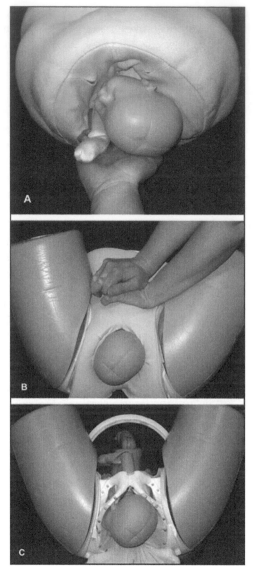

Figure 2.1 Birth training mannequins used for shoulder dystocia training. A. Prototype 2. B. Prototype 3 with skin on. C. Prototype 3 with skin off.

simulation-based training on a central line task trainer, whereas the control group received more traditional bedside training. The authors found a success rate of 51% for first cannulation among the simulation group as opposed to 37% for the control group. The successful CVC insertion rate was 78% for the simulation group compared with 67% for the control group. The simulation training was independently and significantly associated with success at the first cannulation attempt and successful CVC insertion, leaving the authors to conclude that the simulation training was "more effective than traditional training." A similar study by Britt et al.[11] evaluated resident performance of CVC insertion on patients after simulation training using a task trainer versus standard training (apprenticeship model). Again, the authors found that the simulation group had a higher level of performance, with a higher comfort level and ability as well as significantly fewer complications.

With an emphasis on technical skills, the surgical discipline has taken advantage of advances in simulation technology to augment more traditional models of training. Surgical task trainers tend to be expensive; therefore, evidence that the use of such trainers leads to quantifiable improvement helps justify the expense of such modalities. To study the potential benefit of a surgical trainer, Zendejas et al.[12] utilized a simulation-based curriculum with a totally extraperitoneal laparoscopic inguinal hernia repair simulator. Fifty participants were randomly assigned to either the simulation group or the control group. The authors found that the residents who had participated in the simulation training had significantly shorter operative times; they had higher operative performance ratings, and, most importantly, their patients had fewer complications during or after the procedure. Additionally, fewer of the patients undergoing surgery by the simulation-trained residents required overnight stays following their hernia repair. This landmark paper by Zendejas et al. was one of the first to evaluate both patient and learner outcomes of a simulation curriculum and provides strong evidence of the utility of such training in improving patient safety.

Team Training: Simulation to Improve Team Performance and Patient Outcomes

In the healthcare setting, effective communication requires teamwork and collaboration among multiple disciplines, including nurses, physicians, and technicians, and it becomes even more crucial in the midst of an emergency. Studies have shown that effective teamwork improves patient outcomes. Much of the work in the field of communication in high-risk enterprises has its origins in the field of aviation. When the Aerospace Human Factors Research Division of the National Aeronautics and Space Administration reported that the causes of many aviation accidents were due to communication errors, ineffective leadership, and flawed decision-making in crisis situations,[13, 14] the burden of responsibility shifted from individual pilot error to inadequate team performance. This led the way to the development of Cockpit Resource Management (CRM), now more commonly referred to as Crew Resource Management. CRM uses simulation along with structured debriefings and teaches the importance of communication among all team members. Many aspects of CRM have found utility in medical team training.

A study by Andreatta et al.[15] was one of the first to show a positive association between simulation-based team training and improved patient outcomes. In this study, mock codes were called randomly at least once a month, in which all code team members responded as they would in an actual code. Participants included pediatric residents, pediatric intensive care unit (PICU) nurses, pediatric hospitalists, pediatric pharmacists, and pediatric ward nurses. Among other components built into their curriculum, the authors emphasized the identification of a team leader and the use of closed-loop confirmatory communication within the code team. The authors then analyzed survival rates following cardiopulmonary arrests before and after their intervention and found an improvement from 33% to 50% after the integration of the formal mock code program into their training curriculum. Although the authors admit that it is difficult to prove causality, a subanalysis did show that as the number of mock code events increased, so did the incremental increases in survival, suggesting a strong correlation between the two.

Another study showing similar improvements in patient outcomes with the use of simulation in team building comes from work by Knight et al.[16] In a prospective observational study with historical controls, the authors examined the effect of team training via in situ simulation on survival to discharge, as well as team performance (as assessed by adherence to American Heart Association (AHA) resuscitation guidelines) after pediatric in-hospital cardiopulmonary arrest. The code team members consisted of cardiovascular intensivists or PICU attendings, fellows, pediatrics hospitalists, pediatrics residents, nurses, respiratory care providers, and ancillary staff. The intervention group underwent "composite resuscitation" training that included AHA Pediatric Advanced Life Support Course Completion, AHA Basic Life Support Course Completion, familiarization with their roles in a code event, familiarization with and use of an intraosseous drill, familiarization with the location and contents of a pediatric code cart, practice with and education about the new cardiopulmonary resuscitation record and a debriefing tool, and finally, participation with in situ mock codes. After analysis of 183 cardiopulmonary arrest events in 124 patients from the historical controls compared with 64 cardiopulmonary arrest events in 46 patients in the intervention group, the authors found a survival to discharge rate of 60.9% of patients in the intervention group as compared with 40.3% of patients in the historical control group. Furthermore, the analysis of team performance during the code events found improved adherence to AHA resuscitation guidelines. The authors conclude that although simulation training was only a part of the composite training, simulation team training was associated with improved code team performance and improved pediatric survival.

In perhaps the most compelling study of simulation team training and improved patient outcomes, Riley et al.[17] prospectively evaluated the effect of interdisciplinary team training on patient morbidity. The authors conducted the study in three small community hospitals. In the control hospital, no interventions took place. One of the intervention hospitals received only didactic training with the TeamSTEPPS' training program (a teamwork curriculum focusing on leadership, situational monitoring, mutual support, and communication), and the remaining hospital received both the TeamSTEPPS' program and in situ simulation training exercises. In their analysis of perinatal morbidity, the authors found a statistically significant improvement of 37% in morbidity between the preintervention and postintervention periods for the hospital exposed to the simulation program. The authors also found that there were no statistically significant differences in the didactic-only or the control hospital, suggesting that "experiential training is critically important in changing the behavior of practicing professionals."

Summary

No high-risk industry has failed to employ simulation while waiting for indisputable evidence of its utility. Thankfully, the field of medicine has not either. As we have seen, the successful and meaningful implementation of simulation requires scarce resources such as personnel, equipment, time, and money. In today's cost-conscious healthcare environment, it is important to demonstrate the efficacy of such costly interventions. There is now a growing body of literature with well-designed prospective studies that has shown the effectiveness of simulation on patient safety and outcomes.

References

1. Owen H. *Simulation in Healthcare Education: An Extensive History.* Switzerland, Springer International Publishing, 2016.

2. Herzer KR, Rodriguez-Paz JM, Doyle PA, et al. A practical framework for patient care teams to prospectively identify and mitigate clinical hazards. *Joint Commission Journal on Quality and Patient Safety.* 2009;35(2):72–81.

3. Fent G, Blythe J, Farooq O, et al. In situ simulation as a tool for patient safety: A systematic review identifying how it is used and its effectiveness. *BMJ Simulation & Technology Enhanced Learning.* 2015;1(3):103–110.

4. Alfredsdottir H and Bjornsdottir K. Nursing and patient safety in the operating room. *Journal of Advanced Nursing.* 2008;61(1):29–37.

5. Riley W, Davis S, Miller KM, et al. Detecting breaches in defensive barriers using in situ simulation for obstetric emergencies. *Quality & Safety in Health Care.* 2010;19(suppl 3):i53–i56.

6. Wetzel EA, Land TR, Pendergrass TL, et al. Identification of latent safety threats using high-fidelity simulation-based training with multidisciplinary neonatology teams. *Joint Commission Journal on Quality and Patient Safety.* 2013;39(6):268–273.

7. Huang GC, Smith CC, Gordon CE, et al. Beyond the comfort zone: Residents assess their comfort performing inpatient medical procedures. *American Journal of Medicine.* 2006;119(1):71.e17–71.e24.

8. Deering S, Poggi S, Macedonia C, et al. Improving resident competency in the management of shoulder dystocia with simulation training. *Obstetrics & Gynecology.* 2004;103(6):1224–1228.

9. Draycott TJ, Crofts JF, Ash JP, et al. Improving neonatal outcome through practical shoulder dystocia training. *Obstetrics & Gynecology.* 2008;112(1):14–20.

10. Evans LV, Dodge KL, Shah TD, et al. Simulation training in central venous catheter insertion: Improved performance in clinical practice. *Academic Medicine.* 2010;85(9):1462–1469.

11. Britt RC, Novosel TJ, Britt LD, et al. The impact of central line simulation before the ICU experience. *American Journal of Surgery.* 2009;197(4):533–536.

12. Zendejas B, Cook DA, Bingener J, et al. Simulation-based mastery learning improves patient outcomes in laparoscopic inguinal hernia repair: A randomized controlled trial. *Annals of Surgery.* 2011;254(3):502–511.

13. Oriol MD. Crew resource management: Applications in healthcare organizations. *Journal of Nursing Administration.* 2006;36(9):402–406.

14. Helmreich RL, Merritt AC, Wilhelm JA. The evolution of Crew Resource Management in training in commercial aviation. *International Journal of Aviation Psychology.* 1999;9(1):19–32.

15. Andreatta P, Saxton E, Thompson M, et al. Simulation-based mock codes significantly correlate with improved pediatric patient cardiopulmonary arrest survival rates. *Pediatric Critical Care Medicine.* 2011;12(1):33–38.

16. Knight LJ, Gabhart JM, Earnest KS, et al. Improving code team performance and survival outcomes: Implementation of pediatric resuscitation team training. *Critical Care Medicine.* 2014;42(2):243–251.

17. Riley W, Davis S, Miller K, et al. Didactic and simulation nontechnical skills team training to improve perinatal patient outcomes in a community hospital. *Joint Commission Journal on Quality and Patient Safety.* 2011;37(8):357–364.

Chapter

3

Using Human-Centered Design to Create a Safer Anesthesia Workspace

Eliot Grigg and Axel Roesler

The Operating Room as a Design Problem

The design of the anesthesia workspace can have an enormous impact on errors, patient safety, and outcomes. To safely endure the wide variety of surgeries performed today, patients' normal physiologic responses to invasive procedures must be selectively suppressed. This delicate balance requires constant, real-time adjustments to anesthetic techniques and is largely mediated through medications. Unintentional deviations are not well tolerated in this compromised physiologic state. The clinicians in charge of orchestrating this balance are human operators, and their performance is constrained not only by their cognitive and physical capabilities but also by the quality of design of the tools that they use. The fields of Human Factors and Cognitive Psychology provide insight into the psychological and physical aspects that constitute human performance: reasoning, decision-making, attention management, work load, and fatigue. Pushing beyond a provider's limits can result in misinterpretation of the present situation, wrong assessments of the current state, miscalibrated plans, and erroneous actions.[1] A century of research on human performance in high-stakes environments, such as aviation and process control, has rendered a comprehensive picture of what human operators are good at (adaptability and imagination), what their limitations are (precision and vigilance), and how technological systems can support or hobble humans at work.[2, 3]

Good design is often invisible. It enables practitioners to get into a flow, working at a constant pace with great precision, alert to anomalies, and capable of adapting actions to changing contexts by providing the right information, at the right time, in the right way.[4] Poor design ranges from odd to frustrating to dangerous.[5] Well-designed clinical systems can augment and maximize the performance of human actors, whereas poorly designed systems can increase cognitive burdens and provoke mistakes. Human operators are often blamed when complex systems fail, hence the term "human error." According to Don Norman, a leading expert in human-centered design:

> The idea that a person is at fault when something goes wrong is deeply entrenched in society … But in my experience, human error usually is a result of poor design: it should be called system error. Humans err continually; it is an intrinsic part of our nature … Pinning the blame on the person may be a comfortable way to proceed, but why was the system ever designed so that a single act by a single person could cause calamity? Worse, blaming the person without fixing the root, underlying cause does not fix the problem: the same error is likely to be repeated by someone else.[6]

An anesthesiologist is a human operator making decisions in a complex system and enacting those decisions on patients in real time. Each provider may engage in multiple, simultaneous decision loops of gathering data, making decisions, acting upon them, and monitoring the results. To ensure a positive outcome, observations must be accurate, decisions must be appropriate, and actions must align properly with the decisions. How the operator interacts with the world is critical, and those interactions are profoundly influenced by how the surrounding systems are designed. Carefully designed clinical systems that consider how providers interact with information systems, clinical tools, and one another will be instrumental in future patient safety improvements.

Human-Centered Design

In the early years of aviation, as cockpits became increasingly complex, the industry attitude was to select pilots with sufficient aptitude or the "right stuff" to navigate complex systems. Engineers creating mechanical systems were more focused on the individual components than the holistic user experience of the pilot. As plane crashes became increasingly prevalent, it became clear that cockpits were increasingly contending with universal human limitations. Human Factors was created to address these common limitations of ergonomics, attention management, cognitive workload, and working memory.[7] Over the years, the world of design has evolved to be increasingly proactive not only to address limitations but also to optimize human capability. More recently, the concept of human-centered design has emerged that puts human needs, capabilities, and behavior first, then designs to accommodate those needs, capabilities, and ways of behaving.[6] Humans have workload limits, are easily distracted, and rely on mental aids during complex tasks. As cognitive support, the mental aids can take the form of visual representations of mental models such as diagrams, to-do lists, checklists, and other markers in the work setting that create mental structure. Due to inevitable individual biases, a generalized model of how to support understanding and usability of cognitive aids is required, and this is the domain of design.

The term "intuitive" is loosely used to mean "easy to use," but a more formal definition is a system that can be operated effectively without explicit instruction, that is, an instruction manual. To achieve this end, an object must explicitly represent its purpose, capabilities, and limitations to its users. Simple objects, like chairs, do this well. There is little confusion about what a chair is designed to do or how to use it (i.e., where to sit). As systems become increasingly complex, a more formal language between systems and users is necessary, and designing systems to be intuitive becomes more challenging. This can be achieved by using archetypal forms that identify essential components as well as nonverbal formal attributes that highlight control elements, indicate proper directions and limits for movement, and distinguish different elements by shape, size, location, material, and color coding. As a last resort, labels in strategic locations can guide use verbally.

For a system to be intuitive, users must have a clear *understanding* of its purpose, operation, and status, which means that these aspects must be readily *discoverable*. Several design principles help ensure that designers clearly communicate with users through the design of an object. The design of a visual product's features can provide *affordances* and make it clear how an object can be used. Informed by the relationship between the physical attributes of an object and the capabilities of a user, affordances describe what is physically possible.[8, 6] The design of a chair, for example, provides the affordance of "seatability." *Signifiers* indicate where actions should take place. Signifiers can be visual, auditory, or tactile, and a combination of several modalities (visual, audible, tactile) can be used to effectively communicate opportunities for interaction like the buttons on a coffee maker. *Constraints* provide limitations and narrow the range of potential actions. The Pin-Index Safety System is an example of a physical constraint that prevents connecting the wrong gas cylinder to an anesthesia machine. *Feedback* is critical to inform users of the status of a system. Orienting the user, confirming an action, and creating a mental model are all critical outcomes of consistent, accurate feedback. The explanations of the current state of a system and its relation to an anticipated state are the conceptual model, or mental model, that a user brings to the interaction with a product or system in a given situation. Standards, conventions, and expectations are all important elements of this conceptual model. The conceptual model of an interaction with a system is both understanding the system and knowing what to do.

Ultimately, the goal of design is to combine form and function such that what to do and how to do it seem obvious. This is achieved when the design matches the conceptual model of the user who encounters the design. Good design *is* the conceptual model of its use. In retrospect, things that are obvious can easily be taken for granted, but making something obvious from the start can be very challenging. Simplicity is fundamentally beneficial and often overlooked. Simple solutions are generally much harder to achieve than more complex ones because it takes more thought to condense systems down to their essence rather than just hanging functions onto a system, like ornaments.[9] Finally, while interaction design should not be confused with form giving, there is value to the final aesthetic outcome. Objects that are aesthetically pleasing in addition to functional tend to form a better emotional connection with the user.[10] This has been demonstrated by Apple Inc. (Cupertino, CA) with their prominent use of design to elevate computers from desktop workstations to aesthetic mobile products that are present in all aspects of daily life.

Designing for clinical systems faces higher stakes than consumer products, so it is vital that systems are designed for when things go wrong, not just when they go well or as expected. Designers must assume that medical practitioners will use a device incorrectly, and either minimize the impact of errors or make the error obvious, allow for a swift recovery, and create error awareness. This is known as "design for resilience," and it incorporates interactions, procedures, physical products, information systems, and communications in a collaborative work setting that relies heavily on technology.

How to Prevent Errors

Historically, errors have been seen in two ways: (1) the result of individual failings and (2) discreet, isolated events. As the study of safety and error prevention has evolved, the field has come to appreciate the contribution that complex systems make to a series of events that culminate at an error with an individual. The classic paradigm is James Reason's "Swiss Cheese Model," where gaps in multiple preventive measures have to align in order for a mistake to propagate through a system.[11] The field of Resilience Engineering provides frameworks to design for error.[12] We assume that errors will happen, known errors will reoccur, and new errors will reveal unknown territories in the design, making redesign necessary to build resilience into the system. The goal is to mistake-proof multiple steps in a process as robustly as possible in order to prevent gaps from aligning.

Mistake proofing comes in four levels. The highest (Level 1) involves eliminating known errors altogether, which is what traditional engineering solutions are directed at.

Coupling two functions is a popular method: for example, not being able to take a car out of park without applying the brake or automatically stopping a dryer when the door opens. Level 2 is designing work settings so that an error can be detected at the time it occurs: grabbing the wrong vial but then putting it back. Level 3 is designing work settings to reveal anomalies, so that defects can be detected after the error has passed along a system: a second person double-checking an infusion and detecting an error in programming. The fourth and lowest level is all the other cognitive aids employed to make clinical practice safer, such as guidelines and some checklists.

1. Mistake proofing levels[13]
2. Eliminate the error
3. Detect the error
4. Detect the defect
5. Cognitive aids

While higher levels of mistake proofing are preferred, they are not always logistically or financially possible. The goal is to try to design systems with the highest possible or practical level and then continue to look for opportunities to push them higher. Another important consideration is error awareness: While level 1 systems tend to mask errors as they try to eliminate them, levels 2 and 3 embed the possibility of errors into the mindset of practitioners. This has an important effect for the awareness of imminent danger in the operation of the system. The ability to detect errors as they happen in level 2 systems and avert them before they have negative consequences has an important cognitive function: It outlines the boundaries of control in the conceptual model of the task at hand and provides a deeper understanding of the operational context. The design challenge for level 2 systems is to make operations visible for external observers. Besides great effects for training, this externalization approach leads directly to level 3 systems. The secondary check-up that is designed into checklist workflows in level 3 has a similar function: By utilizing think-aloud cross-checks following a to-do list of checkpoints, checklists prompt practitioners to externalize their thought processes and actions and thus make workflows observable in collaborative work so that multiple minds can focus attention on work tasks that are easily skipped under high workload. Checking one's and another's actions implements reflective practice, thinking upon doing as an essential reflection activity that leads to a better understanding of the conceptual models that guide operations and workflows.[14]

Level 1 systems are not always desirable. They work well for smaller components in a larger system such as prefilled medication vials or constrained connectors for gas lines, but unless there is confidence in the robustness of a fully automated control system that manages errors in the background, level 1 approaches to large systems' design tend to render human operators out of the control loop with high costs in systems' safety. High-level accidents in control systems and aviation contexts have illustrated the boundaries of such systems.[15] Learning from these lessons, it is highly questionable that complex anesthesia systems can be made error proof following engineering approaches for equipment. The challenge is to design for error, to support practitioners in coping with mistakes, and to stay in control. Patient safety is the product of a resilient workspace design that makes workflow, operations, and sensemaking observable in order to detect errors before they have unwanted consequences.[15, 16] This can be achieved by the design of cognitive support into the workspace. Cognitive support in the form of standardized layouts, structured workflows, checklists, and communication not only serves as a structure for decision-making, collaborative work, and reflective practice but also forms an effective framework for resilience, training, and documentation of best practices.

Clinical Design in Anesthesia

Over the last 100 years, since the Boyle's machine was invented, steady refinements to the anesthesia machine have helped to prevent errors resulting from anesthetic overdose and errors in provision of adequate oxygenation and ventilation. Being largely a mechanical system of gas delivery, the anesthesia machine is amenable to concrete engineering solutions providing the highest level of error proofing: preventing errors from happening. From the Diameter-Index Safety System to oxygen–nitrous coupling, it is often physically impossible to perform certain errors. Redundant systems and multiple alarms (to detect an error after being committed) provide additional levels of safeguards.

Error prevention from mechanical design peaked decades ago, with most of the innovation in anesthesia machines since then coming in the form of new ventilation modes and more elaborate electronic interfaces. While innovations in other parts of the anesthesia workspace, like laryngeal mask airways or video laryngoscopes, have enhanced clinicians' capabilities, few major advances in patient safety have come along since the new monitoring modalities of pulse oximetry and capnography in the 1980s. Anesthesia Information Management Systems have seen wider implementation over the past decade, but while useful for retrospective analyses, most contribute little to the safety of anesthetized patients during procedures other than some rudimentary reminders.[17] Checklists have certainly helped as cognitive aids, but they are superimposed over preexisting systems and processes that still contain a myriad of built-in failure modes. Even the basic layout of the anesthesia workspace, formally described by an anesthesia task analysis in 1978, has changed little in the last half-century.[18]

The most reliable safety measures remove process steps entirely or make structural changes rendering the incorrect choice physically difficult or impossible. When unleaded gas entered the market in the 1980s, the size of the fuel nozzle changed to make it difficult to put the wrong fuel in the wrong vehicle, and this tradition continues today with diesel. The oxygen–nitrous linkage, whether mechanical or electronic, in anesthesia machines makes it impossible to deliver 100% nitrous. The Diameter-Index Safety System makes connecting the incorrect hose nearly impossible, and color-coding gas lines make connecting the correct line to the correct receptacle more likely.

Unfortunately, such decisive interventions only work in specific circumstances when the options can be definitively constrained. The gas delivery system is relatively simple. There are only three mainline gases in use (oxygen, air, and nitrous oxide); only two are given at any one time, and oxygen is usually one of them. There are only three volatile anesthetics in wide use today; they are given one at a time, and they do not require sterility. This is in part why the anesthesia machine has undergone a variety of engineering upgrades during the past 30 years, while the other half of the anesthesia workspace, devoted to the precise titration of intravenous medications, has seen fewer innovations. Most anesthesia carts in use today are indistinguishable from simple tool chests that can be found at a local hardware store. Some have some basic medication organization capabilities, but they tend to focus on the more mundane, administrative elements of medication handling: inventory, access control, and billing.

One recent effort to eliminate medication errors involves updating small bore connections. Luer-type connections, once a triumph of standardization in the 19th century, have recently become a cross-compatibility liability. Little prevents providers from giving medications intended for enteral or neuraxial routes into an intravenous line. The Global Enteral Device Supplier Association is working on creating separate connections for enteral, neuraxial, respiratory, limb cuff, urethral, and intravenous lines that prevent misconnections (GEDSA, Columbus, OH, USA). While this will help prevent giving a toxic dose of local anesthetic intended for an epidural into an IV, the complexity of intravenous medications has prevented more comprehensive safety design solutions.

Medication Safety in Anesthesia

Anesthesiologists have a unique relationship to the medication cycle because they are the only providers who take complete ownership of the entire process from beginning to end without the benefits of computerized decision support or input from pharmacy that many other providers enjoy. The entire medication cycle is complex and mentally intensive. It includes (1) prescribing, (2) dispensing, (3) preparing, (4) administering, and (5) recording and monitoring. Each one of these steps consists of multiple sub-steps, and each one of those is subject to multiple failure modes. A Failure Modes and Effects Analysis performed at Seattle Children's Hospital (SCH) revealed a total of 19 substeps with 68 possible failure modes in the entire anesthesia medication cycle.[19]

Despite this outsize risk, medication handling in anesthesia relies heavily on provider accuracy and vigilance, both of which inevitably fail. A medium- to large-sized medical center performing 20–30,000 anesthetics a year with an average of 8–10 medications per case, and 15 20 individual administrations could easily have half a million medication administrations in anesthesia. Even with error rates of less than 0.1%, a medical center could reasonably expect a few hundred medication errors (of varying consequence) in the operating room annually.

There are a handful of existing countermeasures designed to address specific vulnerabilities. The ASTM International color-coded standard for medication labels in anesthesia helps to differentiate medication classes. Well-designed labels with high contrast colors, clear fonts, Tall Man lettering, and multiple text orientations can similarly help to identify syringes. Prefilled syringes that take medication vials out of the equation can eliminate six of the medication substeps along with 19 associated potential failure modes. Prefilled syringes are level 1 mistake proofing for vial swaps because they eliminate the vials entirely, which makes them a robust solution. However, they only address a piece of the medication cycle, so other solutions are needed to address additional vulnerabilities.

Example #1 Anesthesia medication trays

At SCH, a team of clinicians and designers created two design-based solutions to help reduce medication errors during anesthesia. In Seattle, medications are stored in a drawer of the anesthesia cart, and providers must select a vial before diluting and transferring to a syringe. Originally, vials were stored all together in the drawer and divided by individual medications. The sections were arranged alphabetically, so similarly sized and shaped vials could be next to one another. Because there is little standardization for vial appearance in the pharmaceutical industry, even within one section there could be several different looking vials. There were over a dozen different types of medications and multiple samples of each type, which meant a drawer of over a hundred individual vials to potentially be confused. This large number also meant that the absence of a few vials could not be appreciated, so it was unclear which vials had been used.

Instead of a whole drawer filled with medications, later the vials were divided into individual patient containers. Fishing tackle boxes were used to organize a sample of vials devoted to an individual patient. At the time, the primary motivation was to facilitate pharmacy billing, but it was an incremental improvement from the giant drawer of medications. Still, this meant around two dozen medications in a single container that were organized alphabetically to facilitate the pharmacy restocking. The vials were standing upright, which meant reading the labels was impossible without removing the vials. Rarely used and potentially dangerous items were next to high use items, and there were no external cues as to the identity of the vial beyond the difficult-to-read label (Figure 3.1).

The final iteration of the medication drawer further divided the medications into five different medication boxes, each designed for single patient use:

1. Primary tray
2. Secondary tray
3. Emergency tray
4. Regional tray
5. Cardiac/transplant tray

The primary tray contains the six most commonly used medications (propofol, lidocaine, cefazolin, ondansetron, ketorolac, and dexamethasone) plus two vials of saline for dilution or reconstitution (Figure 3.2). A laryngeal mask anesthetic in an adult-sized patient uses every vial in the primary tray and nothing else (other than controlled substances). These six medications are also the only medications required in 85% of the operating room cases at SCH, meaning that no other medication tray had to be accessed. As the case progresses and vials are removed, the options decrease and the safety effect increases.

The secondary tray contains the 10 next most commonly used medications (Figure 3.3). This tray contains higher-risk medications like muscle relaxants and vasoactive agents. Because these medications are kept separate, the tray requires intentional access by the provider. Dividing the medications means fewer options within a single tray. The medications in the secondary tray also have more distinctive form factors to help limit confusion. The highest risk medications also live within color-coded wells to further distinguish them. Color-coding was reserved for only two medication classes, muscle relaxants and vasopressors, to maximize the utility of coloring.

Medications used in emergencies or rarely, typically in less than 1% of cases, were placed in an emergency tray. These included drugs for allergic reactions or cardiopulmonary resuscitation. The form factor of this tray prevented much in the way of specific layout design, but some of the medications, epinephrine and atropine, were stored in cardboard boxes to distinguish them from vials.

A specialized tray was also formulated for regional anesthesia so that local anesthetics used in nerve blocks would not be confused with other medications destined for intravenous lines. Another specialized tray was devised for the more specialized cardiac and transplant teams that supplied more vasoactive substances, heparin or protamine, and bicarbonate. This group of medications would help facilitate care for more complex cases but would rarely be needed outside of the transplant or cardiac context.

Using trays segregated medications to areas where they are needed and removed them from places they are not. Of note, none of the above trays contained controlled substances. For security and accountability reasons, all controlled substances are managed in separate secure boxes assigned to individual providers.

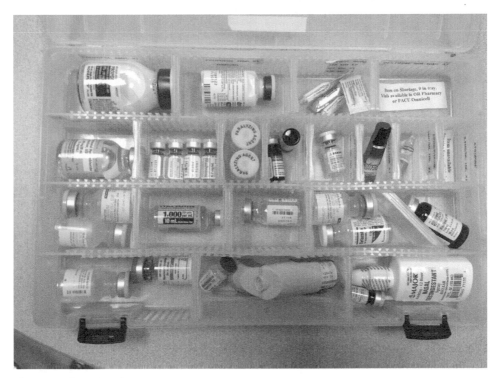

Figure 3.1 Original medication tray
(A black and white version of this figure will appear in some formats. For the color version, refer to the plate section.)

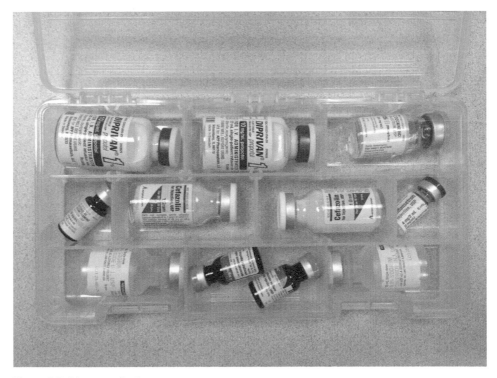

Figure 3.2 Primary medication tray
(A black and white version of this figure will appear in some formats. For the color version, refer to the plate section.)

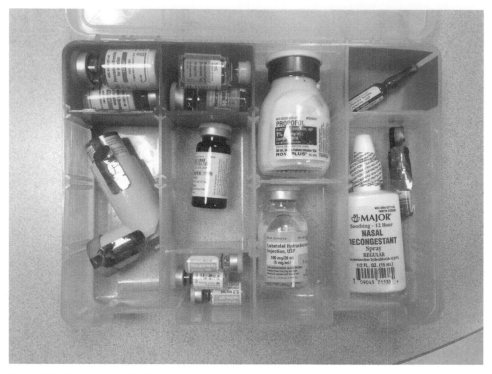

Figure 3.3 Secondary medication tray
(A black and white version of this figure will appear in some formats. For the color version, refer to the plate section.)

The medication trays were designed around several design principles:

1. Separation
2. Constraint
3. Orientation
4. Signifiers

Separation. Instead of a single medication tray with numerous choices, the medication vials are separated between different trays. While the separation creates a series of different medication trays, each of which has to be tracked and stocked, it allows providers to partition the medications by various criteria. Some are divided according to specific clinical applications like cardiac surgery or regional anesthesia. Others are partitioned by the frequency of use. If the secondary tray is only accessed for 15% of cases, the opportunity to confuse certain medications (like the powdered forms of cefazolin and vecuronium) is reduced by 85%. It also allows any given tray to have fewer similar-looking vials; for example, the myriad number of 1- to 2-mL vials. Separation between trays creates a concrete, physical barrier that is effective at preventing vial confusion. Less definitive but also helpful is the physical separation of similar vials within a single tray. The small vials of ondansetron, dexamethasone, and ketorolac are placed on opposite ends of the tray to differentiate them.

Constraint. One of the primary benefits of separating medications is that it allows providers to focus on fewer medications within a specific tray. The likelihood of confusion goes up exponentially with each medication that is added to a specific area of focus, so the fewer medications available in one area, the better. When accessing the primary tray, only seven different medications are available. Such a constrained set of options is much easier to navigate because an operator can reasonably be expected to keep five to seven items in a mental model, while a dozen is too many. Of course, too few medications could prevent providers from having necessary tools available, so there is a limit constraint.

With a finite number of overall medications, the more medications are separated into different trays, the more constrained the options become within a single tray. However, there are limits to this trend. Too many trays begin to create problems similar to those that arise when there are too many medications within a single tray. The goal is to strike a balance between parsing medications so that the number of trays and the number of medications within a tray is in the single digits. George Miller's oft-cited paper from 1956 suggests that the number of objects the average human can keep in working memory is 7 ± 2.[20] The system at SCH ended up with five different trays with seven to ten medications per tray.

Orientation. In addition to separating medications within each tray, there are other ways of minimizing confusion within trays. Duplicate vials are placed symmetrically to reinforce a mental model of organization. Symmetrical patterns are easier to remember than arbitrary or alphabetical arrangements. Vials are placed horizontally so that the labels are readable without removing them from the wells.

Signifiers. Some of the wells within the trays are color-coded as an additional indicator of which types of medications are contained within. The colors match the ASTM medication class standard, but, significantly, only a few important colors are used to maximize their impact: red for muscle relaxants and violet for vasopressors. Having medications come in different preparations can also help to differentiate them: vials, prefilled syringes, bags for light protection or commercial preparations in boxes. Interestingly, signifiers on the medication vials themselves proved less useful. Given the complexities of pharmaceutical supply chains in the United States, it was impossible to always stock identical-looking vials for each medication, let alone to control the visual content of the medication labels, so the design team de-emphasized the actual labels on the vials and focused more on surrounding signifiers to aid in correct identification.

Dividing the medication trays of high-use items also had other efficiency benefits. An entire day's worth of trays could be stocked into a single cart, which decreased the need for constant restocking. This made it more likely that providers had the necessary medications available throughout the day. By segregating low-use medications, fewer had to be stocked in each anesthetizing location, which ended up saving tens of thousands of dollars in pharmacy inventory and waste per year. The design effort was focused on minimizing vial swaps; however, for administration, medications must be prepared and stored in syringes, which pose an analogous swap risk.

Example #2 Anesthesia medication template

Once medications are prepared in syringes, they are placed atop the anesthesia cart or machine, waiting to be utilized at different points throughout a procedure. Some syringes are used once, some more than once, and others not at all. Selecting a syringe seems like a trivial task in isolation, but with the stress, unpredictability, and repetition of the operating room, after tens of thousands of such actions, mistakes will occur. The Anesthesia Medication Template (AMT) was designed as a repository for medication syringes during a procedure (Figure 3.4). In addition to minimizing inadvertent syringe swaps, the design goals of the AMT include: (1) to diminish the search time and overall cognitive load on clinicians selecting syringes, (2) to exploit blank spaces, and (3) to standardize the medication layout in all anesthetizing locations within an institution.

The AMT relies on similar design principles to the medication trays: separation, orientation, constraint, and signifiers. The primary difference is that the layout and contents of

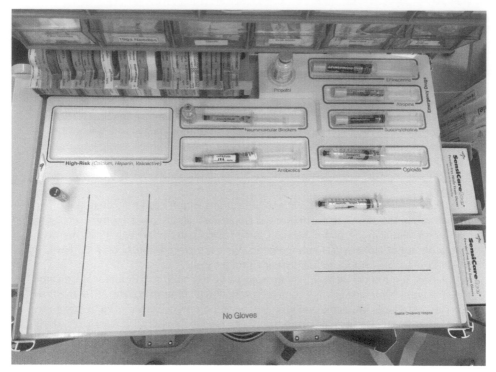

Figure 3.4 Anesthesia medication template
(A black and white version of this figure will appear in some formats. For the color version, refer to the plate section.)

the medication trays are known a priori, and they are primarily accessed during setup for the case, a more controlled environment. The AMT is a much more dynamic tool used continuously throughout a case, and the specific contents may be different for each procedure. The AMT is divided into two sections: an area with drug class–specific cells designed to accommodate individual syringes and a freeform workspace for medication preparation or other unanticipated needs.

The medication template was created with similar design principles to the trays:

1. Simplicity
2. Separation
3. Signifiers
4. White space
5. Mental model

Simplicity. The first design question is, Which drug classes receive dedicated cells? The temptation is to create an indented space or well for every drug class or for the most commonly used medications, but this creates two problems: (1) the increased visual clutter dilutes the efficacy of individual cells and (2) the consequent loss of free space within a finite area reduces the flexibility of the device. The goal was not to accommodate the most commonly used medications but rather to risk-stratify a subset of problematic ones in order to create the fewest dedicated syringe cells as possible while remaining effective.

If the likelihood of confusing a particular medication is high, or if the consequences of confusing a medication are severe, then the medication deserves a dedicated space in a standardized template. Due to its distinctive white color, propofol is unlikely to be confused with other medications, so it does not require a specific space. The consequences of accidentally administering muscle relaxants, however, can be severe, so a space is warranted for them. To further push simplicity, if two medications are often confused or always used in a pair (like reversal agents), then only one of the two agents may need to be given a distinct location in order to segregate the two.

Like many design projects, the first few iterations of the AMT were much more complex than the final product. The iterative design process was largely an exercise in restraint to distill the device down to its simplest, most useful form.

The final template for general pediatric anesthesia included the following dedicated spaces:

1. Epinephrine
2. Atropine
3. Succinylcholine
4. Opioids
5. Muscle relaxants
6. Antibiotics
7. Miscellaneous "High Risk"

The first three are emergency medications that are not needed routinely and are given additional segregation. The last area is a more general "miscellaneous" area for a variety of high-risk medications including heparin, calcium, and vasoactive medications, such as ephedrine or phenylephrine. This leaves only three routine medication classes – opioids, muscle relaxants, and antibiotics – as the primary ones selected for specific areas. Many routinely administered but lower-risk medications, such as antiemetics, steroids, or non-steroidal anti-inflammatories, do not require special areas on the template. None of the sedative or hypnotics have dedicated spaces. The original version had all of the elements. After multiple iterations and revisions, this was the simplest constellation of elements the design team settled on for general pediatric cases.

A second pediatric cardiac/liver template kept all of the above spaces in the same location but added spaces dedicated to:

1. A second epinephrine concentration
2. Phenylephrine
3. Calcium

It was important to keep as much of the original design as possible because providers often move between roles and may use multiple versions of the template. As such, most of the template should look familiar from one room to the next, and any medication with a dedicated space must be in the same arrangement from one version to the next. Succinylcholine, for example, can't appear different or move around in different versions of the template. At the same time, the goal is to have the fewest versions of the template as possible, which is why the only other template at SCH is the combined cardiac/liver layout. The transplant and cardiac groups were combined into a single layout, which is also used in the interventional cardiology suites. No third version was allowed.

Separation. Much like the medication trays, separation is a powerful physical and visual tool to differentiate medications. Syringes in similar medication classes, like succinylcholine and nondepolarizing neuromuscular blockers, are physically separated in the medication trays. Syringes that are used infrequently but are high-risk, like emergency medications, have special separation on an elevated platform at the back of the template. More commonly used medications are toward the front, nearer to the provider.

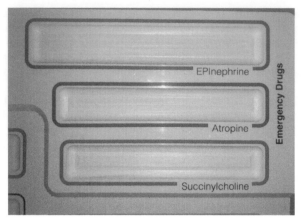

Figure 3.5 Color and background detail. *Original photos by Eliot Grigg and Figures 3.2 and 3.3 by Sally Rampersad; photos taken at Seattle Children's Hospital which did not require permission for their use.* (A black and white version of this figure will appear in some formats. For the color version, refer to the plate section.)

Signifiers. Using multiple cues increases the reliability of identifying individual syringes. Cues may be visual, auditory, or tactile, and there is some evidence that using different senses at the same time (audio and visual) helps to communicate more information without overwhelming a single sensory input. The existing medication template only employed visual cues, but it used a variety of different dimensions to ensure proper syringe identification. When scanning a workspace, there is a hierarchy of how the brain locates a target:[21]

Location → Color → Shape → Text

The location in the two-dimensional plane is the first clue to identifying a syringe. More commonly used syringes are toward the front and less common ones toward the back. Emergency syringes, rarely used but essential when needed, occupy an elevated platform that distinguishes them in three-dimensional space.

Color is the next most obvious clue. The colored outlines of the syringe cells match the ASTM standard. To maximize its effectiveness, color must be used sparingly so it only occupies a thin outline rather than a completely filled background (Figure 3.5). Having as few colors as possible also reinforces the restraint needed when choosing the number and drug classes to occupy dedicated cells. The basic pediatric template uses only four colors (violet, red, green, and blue) plus black and white. All of the colors are highly saturated and contrast well with the white background of the template. The white background also works well with syringes filled with transparent fluids where the background can be seen through the syringe and can affect the reading of the label.

Most of the syringes are of similar shape; however, size can be a differentiator. Using a variety of standard syringe sizes ranging from 1 mL to 60 mL can help distinguish specific medications. Size can also help distinguish differences within a single-colored medication class. For example, fentanyl can be placed in a 5-mL syringe, while morphine can be placed in a 10-mL syringe. Overall, the general shape and texture of the syringes is largely determined by manufacturers and remains mostly uniform.

Finally, the text, or label, is usually the last signifier that the brain will interpret because it requires visual clarity in the center of the visual field, sustained focus, and engagement of the language centers in the brain. The text is the most specific clue to the contents of the syringe but is by no means a foolproof way of communicating with providers. The font, color, size, spacing, and location all matter in terms of placing text. Short labels with lowercase sans serif fonts are the easiest to read quickly. The syringes also sit horizontally to make the labels easier to read, even though a vertical orientation would allow for more syringes to fit in a smaller space.

White Space. Unoccupied areas can also communicate information. While antibiotics are generally low-risk medications, having a dedicated cell that may be unoccupied can serve as a reminder that the medication has not been given. An empty space for emergency medications serves as a reminder that they have not been prepared. The unadorned free space is also important. To achieve standardization, the template must be versatile, but it is impossible to anticipate every case. The flexible workspace nearest the provider allows users to accommodate larger syringes, other syringes, or medication preparation supplies to ensure the template can be used for a variety of cases. Building flexibility into the space by not prescribing every inch of the template helps users accept and adapt to the device.

Mental model. The relationship of the cells to one another helps to direct the eye while it scans the template, and aligning orthogonal edges helps to create a fluid, coherent mental model of the template layout. After using the template for a while, a user will create a mental map of the syringe locations, which is why having a standard layout is critical for multiple sites within an institution where providers work in teams or change locations. Concerns have been raised that creating such "mental shortcuts" with a template may prevent users from closely scrutinizing syringes, but the combination of multiple cues to identify syringes helps to mitigate that effect. Overall, the design team felt that the benefits of a standardized layout far outweighed the risk of introducing mental shortcuts.

The Data

Employing all of this design theory in the clinical space is relatively untested in the medication-handling sphere, so it was important to measure the impact of the interventions in a real clinical space. In a simulated environment with well-controlled circumstances, utilization of the AMT reduced the incidence of medication dosing errors by almost 80%.[22] Over the course of a two-year study in the operating room at SCH, the mean monthly error rate for all reported medication errors decreased from 1.24 to 0.65 errors per 1,000 anesthetics, while the mean monthly error rate specific to swap, preparation, miscalculation, and timing errors (the ones more directly related to the template) decreased from 0.97 to 0.35 errors per 1,000 anesthetics.[22]

Measuring medication errors is challenging. Self-reporting, the typical standard, is fraught with recall bias and undoubtedly misses some errors. Direct observation is resource-intensive and often unsustainable over the long periods of time required to capture these relatively rare events. Operating rooms are complex environments with many confounding factors. Despite all of these potential issues, the dramatic impact of the template is compelling. The effects of the template, the trays, and a few other targeted interventions, like an infusion checklist and better access to labels, resulted in years of sustained reduction in medication errors.[19]

Cognitive Artifacts and Future Directions

The overall goal of bringing design principles to the operating room is to extend and enhance human capabilities by accounting for innate human limitations and implanting "knowledge in the world." As Don Norman observes:

> The power of the unaided mind is highly overrated … Unaided memory, thought, and reasoning are all limited in power … The real powers come from devising external aids that enhance cognitive abilities … through the development of tools of thought – cognitive artifacts – that … strengthen mental powers.[6]

Placing knowledge in the world relieves providers of the burden of maintaining too much knowledge in their heads.[6, 23] Making knowledge external and accessible to multiple providers helps facilitate shared mental models.[24] Embedding clues on how to use and maximize clinical objects helps to guide clinicians in real time and prevents errors resulting from human–machine interaction. Accounting for inherent human limitations, whether they be biases within the visual system or cognitive limitations like working memory, helps to enhance human abilities.

One of the benefits of employing standardization, organization, and visual cues is that it decreases the cognitive load on providers while identifying medications. Decreasing cognitive load can not only increase the accuracy of syringe or vial selection in a distracting or repetitive environment, but it may also have downstream effects on other cognitive processes. For example, there is some evidence that the medication template can decrease the incidence of calculation errors.[22] When mental bandwidth is freed up for other tasks, providers can spend more effort on making clinical decisions.

The attributes of good clinical design are:

1. *Simple*: employ the least complex solution possible
2. *Intuitive*: require little or no training
3. *Error proof*: make it difficult to use something incorrectly
4. *Permitting*: help improve performance rather than just prevent errors
5. *Aesthetic*: create an emotional connection to the user

Good design requires tremendous discipline. The temptation is always to add complexity to solutions for complex problems. A much more difficult challenge is to distill a problem and its solution to its essence. Robust solutions make errors near-impossible without creating impediments to normal clinical flow. For example, prefilled syringes eliminate vial swaps entirely because all of the error-prone steps involved in vial preparation are removed, yet the clinician is not adversely affected.

In addition to organizing the workspace and redesigning the visual, tactile, and auditory attributes of clinical tools, a large opportunity for future design will come from systems integration. Infusion pumps, electronic health records, medication carts, and vaporizers will someday need to coordinate with one another. Communication between the various anesthesia tools will allow for more automation and further offload the provider to focus on more human-centric skills like problem-solving and creative thinking. The medication workspace specifically would benefit from a more integrated solution because current processes are very manual and error-prone. In the early days of anesthesia, providers had to prepare and physically administer volatile anesthetics, but now they are able to simply dial a concentration into a machine and also, exhaled concentrations can be measured. Perhaps someday a similar solution will be available for intravenous medications. There are enormous opportunities to bring the lessons and expertise from interactive design to the clinical arena. By understanding human factors and limitations and thoughtfully organizing the clinical workspace and redesigning clinical tools, there are numerous opportunities to enhance clinician performance and to improve patient safety.

References

1. Proctor RW and Van Zandt T. *Human Factors in Simple and Complex Systems*, 2nd ed., Boca Raton, Taylor & Francis Group, 2008.

2. Salas E, Jentsch F, and Maurino, D, eds. *Human Factors in Aviation*, 2nd ed., Burlington, Academic Press, 2010.

3. Kosslyn SM. Aspects of a cognitive neuroscience of mental imagery. *Science*. 1988;240:1621–1626.

4. Lidwell W, Holden K, and Butler J. *Universal Principles of Design*. Beverly, Rockport, 2010.

5. Leveson NG and Turner CS. An investigation of the Therac-25 accidents. *IEEE Computer*. 1993;26:18–41.

6. Norman DA. *The Design of Everyday Things: Revised and Expanded Edition*. New York, Basic Books, 2013.

7. Guastello SJ. *Human Factors Engineering and Ergonomics: A Systems approach*. 2nd ed., Boca Raton, Taylor & Francis, 2014.

8. Gibson JJ. *The Ecological Approach to Visual Perception*. Hillsdalen, Lawrence Erlbaum Associates Inc., 1986.

9. Gallo C. *The Innovation Secrets of Steve Jobs: Insanely Different Principles for Breakthrough Success*. New York, McGraw-Hill, 2011.

10. Norman DA. *Emotional Design: Why We Love (or Hate) Everyday Things*. New York, Basic Books, 2004.

11. Reason J. *Human Error*. Cambridge, Cambridge University Press, 1990.

12. Paries J, Wreathall J, and Hollnagel E, eds., *Resilience Engineering in Practice: A Guidebook*. Boca Raton, Taylor & Francis, 2011.

13. Tsuda Y. Implications of foolproofing in the manufacturing process. *Quality through Engineering Design*. Kuo W., ed., New York, Elsevier, 1993.

14. Degani A, Wiener EL. On the design of flight deck procedures. NASA Ames Research Center. NASA Contractor Report 177642, 1994.

15. Klein G, Moon B, and Hoffman RF. Making sense of sensemaking I: Alternative perspectives. *IEEE Intelligent Systems*. 2006a;21:70–73.

16. Klein G, Moon B, and Hoffman RF. Making sense of sensemaking II: A macrocognitive model. *IEEE Intelligent Systems*. 2006b;21:88–92.

17. Stonemetz J and Ruskin K, eds. *Anesthesia Informatics*. London, Springer-Veralong, 2008.

18. Drui AB, Behm RJ, and Martin WE. Predesign investigation of the anesthesia operational environment. *Anesthesia & Analgesia*. 1973;52:584–591.

19. Martin LD, Grigg E, and Verma S, et al. Outcomes of a failure mode and effects analysis for medication errors in pediatric anesthesia. *Pediatric Anesthesia*. 2017;27:571–580.

20. Miller GA. The magical number seven, plus or minus two: Some limits on our capacity for processing information. *Psychological Review*. 1956;63:81–97.

21. Treisman A. Features and objects: The fourteenth Bartlett memorial lecture. *The Quarterly Journal of Experimental Psychology*. 1988;40A:201–237.

22. Grigg E, Martin L, Ross F, et al. Assessing the impact of the anesthesia medication template on medication errors during anesthesia: A prospective study. *Anesthesia & Analgesia*. 2017;124:1617–1625.

23. Hutchins E. *Cognition in the Wild*. Cambridge, MA, MIT Press, 1995.

24. Zhang J and Norman DA. Representations in distributed cognitive tasks. *Cognitive Science*. 1994;18:87–122.

Preoccupation with Failure: Daily Management System

Chapter 4

Aaron C. Dipzinski and Lynn D. Martin

Introduction

Throughout the spectrum of the healthcare experience, a patient moves across several intricate systems. Often these systems are disjointed. The complexity of this delivery system routinely places healthcare providers and staff in high-risk situations. High reliability organizations (HROs) offer insight into managing an environment with persistent risk.

Behavior within an HRO is characterized by five consistent actions: "(1) tracks small failures, (2) resists oversimplification, (3) remains sensitive to operations, (4) maintains capabilities for resilience, and (5) takes advantage of shifting locations of expertise."[1] There is an emphasis on the preoccupation with failure with the detection of small failures or near misses. These near misses provide insight to potential or real system failures and also aim to anticipate and identify significant areas of risk.[1] A Daily Management System (DMS)[2] serves as a structure that aligns with the five characteristics of an HRO.

A DMS is a systematic approach that improves business operations in healthcare via identification and elimination of nonvalue added (waste) activities (Figure 4.1). Providers and staff are encouraged to develop problem-solving capacity and continuous improvement across an organization.[2] An organization's daily actions are predictable patterns of behavior necessary to achieve consistent and highly reliable operations, which ultimately promote safe operations for patients and staff.

The DMS has nine key components supported by Leader Standard Work (LSW).

1. Continuous improvement
2. Visual management
3. Data trending and analysis
4. Performance management
5. Process standard work
6. Standard work validation
7. Version control
8. Problem escalation and response
9. Ideas for improvement

The DMS operates in the context of a larger organizational management system. Leadership routines are critical to provide for a DMS. A leader's work, in turn, is directed by the core principles and strategy direction of the organization.

The entirety of the management system includes three aspects of organizational behavior: (1) strategic development, (2) implementation of projects and initiatives, and (3) man-

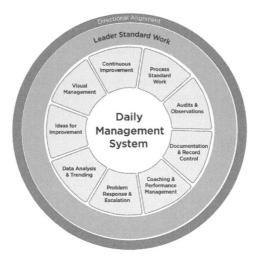

Figure 4.1 Daily management system. The DMS is a set of operational patterns practiced daily. Leader standard work envelops the routines, illustrating the importance of leadership routines to support an effective DMS.
(A black and white version of this figure will appear in some formats. For the color version, refer to the plate section.)

agement of daily operations. Organizations exhibiting a preoccupation with failure hold safety as a core value throughout the strategic planning process and prioritization activities. These principles are woven into the fabric of the management system.

Leader Standard Work (LSW): Starting with the Leader

LSW refers to predictable, repeatable routines that leaders follow. This management practice allows leaders to focus on abnormal conditions, on the development of team members, and on problem identification and solutions. Effective LSW is documented and visible to all team members. LSW includes the following six elements:

1. Regular presence where the care is delivered: Walking all aspects of the clinical sites of care. Clear visual tools are used to identify normal from abnormal conditions.
2. Rounding for influence: Intentional and visible conversations to reinforce safety and other cultural imperatives and behaviors as core values.
3. Attendance and attention: Presence at huddles where key performance metrics are displayed and reviewed.
4. Developing self and others: Training, coaching, and encouraging the philosophy of problem identification and improvement.
5. Escalation path and response: Timely processing and communicating the resolution of identified issues.
6. Accountability: Use of visual boards to track key processes and outcome measures as well as alert leaders to areas of opportunity to provide support for all team members.

In order to develop meaningful LSW, a leader starts with the question, "What are my current actions that advance clinical operations, support management, and improve patient safety?" Those activities should be incorporated into LSW routines, along with new actions that will also advance the DMS and improve patient safety. The ultimate objective for LSW is to create an environment where team members feel empowered to escalate concerns and improve the methods for delivering safe care. The approach, the attitude, and the way the leader deploys standard work determine whether an organization, department, or unit achieves the desired culture. LSW promotes consistency with clear expectations and direction. When paired with enthusiasm and encouragement, teams can excel.

Visual Management

Visual management[3] is the outward expression of operational status, organizational focus, and a unique cultural identity through the display of measures and visual indicators that convey the story of operations and organizational values. Effective visual management resides in all aspects of the workplace and is used to promote action by the teams. It drives action by linking the actual status of operations to a desired state or target. A visual workplace aims to expose problems through open and meaningful messaging. Examples include graphs displaying data of department measures, indicators displaying information for par levels of supplies that trigger ordering before reaching a critically low level of inventory, or illustrations guiding individuals as to where instrumentation or equipment resides.[3]

Visual management enables an environment of continuous improvement by focusing all team members on solving issues that could increase safety risks. More importantly, visual management provides direction and coaching to the team in the absence of the leader. The DMS operates from the assumption that people intrinsically desire collaboration and will improve in an environment where autonomy exists, information is readily available, and celebration of improvement is a regular occurrence.

For visual management to work, there must be encouragement and reward for showing and knowing the truth of operations.

One place to begin experimenting with visual management tools is in areas where current safety work is already occurring and the information is readily available, such as operational performance metrics or supply chain requirements. As the adoption of this method of management spreads, individuals will often ask for updates, reports, or other forms of communication.

Problem Escalation and Response

An important tenet of the DMS is that anyone has the ability and authority to raise a safety concern. Problem escalation and response should be easy without structural or cultural barriers.

Daily huddle activity consists of a tiered huddle structure. The day starts with a review of operational conditions, with emphasis on areas of high risk, operational challenges, or any variable introducing risk into the area. Issues identified in the frontline huddle move swiftly and progressively through the chain of command for awareness and problem resolution. These issues are reported to senior leadership within a few hours from the first frontline huddles.

Operations conclude the day with a huddle involving the same frontline care teams that started the day. The intent of the end-of-day huddle is a reflection on the planned (morning huddle) versus actual (the status of the day) performance, which helps identify gaps in performance and generate ideas for further improvement and group problem-solving. Ideas are either immediately acted upon or captured for future improvement activities. Assignment of an owner and date is appropriate for issues that will need longer term resolution. Stop-the-line issues are significant safety concerns and require immediate resolution. Other concerns require reporting at the end-of-day huddle, but operations can continue while the issue is reviewed and resolved. Problem escalation and response leads to risk identification, appropriate resource allocation, and improvement.

Performance Management: Clear Expectations and Accountability

The elements of daily performance management are: (1) standard work for leaders and team members, (2) visual controls or visual management, (3) daily accountability (team huddle and improvement routines), and (4) teamwork, including team discipline and accountability to self and to each other. Together, these four elements of individual performance enable high-performing teams to accomplish extraordinary results.

Standard work provides a structure and routine for leaders and team members. When standards exist and are followed, abnormal results and problems are more quickly and easily identified. This practice allows leaders and team members to focus on the abnormal rather than the normal conditions. Visual controls are an important enabler for standard work. Teamwork emphasizes that everyone is accountable for following standards, so that the system can function normally. Continuous improvement is an essential aspect of an individual's performance and may be included in annual goal setting and performance review.

The daily activities of the management system promote the ongoing development and evaluation of each team member. A supervisor's LSW focuses on investment in an individual through consistent, formal coaching routines. Coaching patterns serve as an opportunity to gauge an individual's commitment, while offering a safe forum for feedback. This allows the supervisor and the employee to remain aligned on performance expectations.

Process Standard Work (PSW)

PSW is the steps, sequence, and time required for a process to achieve a specific outcome. Standard daily tasks and responsibilities, which are predictable and repeatable, are the outcome of PSW. As with LSW, PSW is recorded and visible for all who participate in the process. Effective standard work illustrates the best current practice and time of each step in the process, often using pictures to display the actual work method. PSW is vital to a highly reliable organization.

Standard work serves two central purposes. First, PSW is the cornerstone of continuous improvement. The creation of PSW serves as a baseline from which the Plan-Do-Check-Act (PDCA) cycle is applied to continually evolve and improve best practice. The PDCA cycle, or Deming cycle, encapsulates the scientific method and is described in detail in Chapter 5. Second, PSW reduces variation within a process. Lessening variation allows a team to easily distinguish a planned versus actual process outcome. This enables quick escalation and timely root cause identification for processes producing abnormal conditions.

Creating PSW requires observing the current process in real time to capture actual data. This information establishes the process steps, sequence, and time required for the current state or baseline. It is often helpful to have several members collect data, thereby allowing verification of information and building of consensus for PSW. During the observation phase, it is likely that unwanted or unnecessary steps or actions will be identified. This type of activity is commonly referred to as "waste." Waste is any motion or communication within a process that is unnecessary (nonvalue added) from the perspective of the patient or internal customer. It is estimated that up to 95% of healthcare processes consist of nonvalue added activity. Consequently, when documenting PSW, the primary focus is on removing this identified waste.

The creation and adoption of PSW is challenging to implement. Often, long-held performance patterns that are ingrained in the process need to change. One approach is to introduce the foundational thinking of a DMS; specifically, standardization is to start with "5S" methodology. This practice suggests a sequence of activities teams follow to organize and standardize the workplace. These activities are:

- **Sort**: remove all items from the workplace that are not needed. The aim of sorting is to clearly distinguish required from preferential, outdated, or surplus items.
- **Straighten**: organize needed instruments, equipment, supplies, or other items throughout the workplace. Identifying and labeling are included in this phase with the aim that anyone, even those unfamiliar with the area, could find and replace the item. The outcome ensures that necessary items are in the correct place and allows for effortless and immediate retrieval.
- **Shine**: this phase highlights the physical appearance of any item and the workplace itself. Emphasis is placed on removing waste and dirt. This routine builds pride and professionalism within the team. It promotes safety, of which clean instruments, equipment, and physical workspace are the foundation.
- **Standardize**: this phase ensures the method is owned, documented, and visual to all team members. This phase provides the basis for the PDCA cycle and for sustainability.
- **Sustain**: the aim of this phase is to maintain the tangible and cultural gains resulting from the prior work. To accomplish this objective, frequent process validation routines are utilized.

The 5S process is a visual control system for organizing and maintaining department work areas. In the final state, it is easy to identify where all clinical equipment and instrumentation reside throughout the entire healthcare facility.

As with PSW, sustainability of 5S requires an embedded practice. Improvement, validation, and review of PSW is a daily routine in order to prevent entropy of culture and work routines.

Process Standard Work Validation – A System of Sustainment

The foundation of a sustainable process is constant monitoring, especially when the process is first adopted. Daily observation (auditing) of the process provides opportunities for real-time feedback regarding the effectiveness of the standard work. Routine observation serves as an important reinforcement to follow standard work and an opportunity to learn about any challenges with the current standards. Using terms such as "validation" or "confirmation" rather than "auditing" may be less intimidating and better accepted by frontline workers (Figure 4.2).

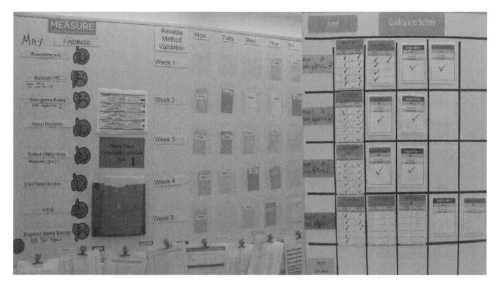

Figure 4.2 Standard work validation. This illustration provides two examples of a standard work validation method. Both examples communicate that the processes are part of the current validation, the status of the actual validation, and the results of observations.
Legends and figures supplied by Aaron Dipzinski, photos taken at Seattle Children's Hospital which did not require permission for their use.
(A black and white version of this figure will appear in some formats. For the color version, refer to the plate section.)

Visual tools are used to make expectations clear as well as to illustrate whether or not observations are complete or if measures are on track to meet their targets. Observations may be made by a leader or area manager, but as the process becomes more established, frontline workers may take on this role as the process begins to become self-sustaining.

Data Trending

Management systems are dependent upon accurate data to detect areas of operational risk. Further, proper analytics afford teams the ability to visualize results, determine the outcomes of prior experimentation, and direct future action by guiding prioritization.

Ideas for Improvement – Capturing the Collective Genius

Ideas for improvement *can* come from anyone within the organization and *must* come from the frontline. Huddles are typically done once or twice daily. They offer a forum to solicit ideas for improvement and celebrate the completion of improvement projects.

Collective awareness of improvement ideas is often achieved with a visibility board, which may include the display of past, present, and proposed improvements.

Continuous improvement is an iterative process with many small changes leading to a significant impact on outcomes over time. Through experience, practice, and a constant focus on observation of the frontline process where the value-added work occurs, the culture adapts into one that embraces quick "point improvement" and rapid tests of change. As team members become more comfortable offering suggestions for improvement, the DMS will rely heavily on visual management to support the multiple ideas for improvement. The department will also need to establish a version control process to avoid confusion.

Version Control

Version control is a subtle routine within the DMS. The purpose of this practice is to ensure that there is a reliable method to post the current version of work methods, protocols, LSW, metrics, tools, checklists, visual controls, organizational goals, and any other document individuals or teams rely on to focus attitudes and behaviors in their daily work. It is paramount for a safe environment that care teams are working from the latest version of any guideline that determines their work methods.

Conclusion

The complexity of the healthcare delivery system routinely places healthcare providers and staff in high-risk situations. An effective DMS uses the five essential characteristics of HROs[1] and ensures that these essential principles of high reliability are built into daily operations. The prevailing mindset embedded within the DMS is a preoccupation with failure and a desire to make problems visible, identify root causes, and test countermeasures. Improvements in one area will often uncover a safety risk in another area, so the DMS is perpetually evolving and changing to meet the next challenge.

References

1. Weick KE and Sutcliffe KM. *Managing the Unexpected: Resilient Performance in an Age or Uncertainty*. 2nd ed., Hoboken, NJ, Jossey-Bass, 2007.

2. Maurer M, Canacari E, Eng K, et al. Building a culture of continuous improvement and employee engagement using a daily management system part 1: Overview. *Journal of Nursing Administration*. March 2018;48(3):127–131.

3. Maurer M, Browall P, Phelan C et al. Continuous improvement and employee engagement, part 2, design, implementation and outcomes of a daily management system. *Journal of Nursing Administration*. April 2018;48(4):209–215.

Chapter

5

Lean versus Model for Improvement

Julianne Mendoza and David Buck

The science of Quality Improvement (QI) originated from pioneers such as W. Edwards Deming, Joseph Juran, and Walter Shewhart. Deming's work can be summarized by his "system of profound knowledge" which consists of four key elements: appreciation for a system, understanding variation, a theory of knowledge, and psychology.[1] From these common origins, different frameworks for improvement subsequently developed. More recently, the Institute for Healthcare Improvement has been instrumental in shaping this work to apply to the healthcare industry. The two most commonly used QI methodologies in healthcare are Lean and the Model for Improvement (MFI). Lean originated from the work of Toyota with a focus on production systems, reducing waste, and standardized work. The MFI is a general interactive approach for learning from experience and turning knowledge into action. Both are data-driven approaches to continuous improvement and offer a practical approach to applying the principles of QI to a healthcare project.[2]

It may be beneficial to adopt a primary framework for learning improvement, particularly when starting out. This helps to create a uniform culture and understanding around QI work at your institution. However, both methodologies are based on similar principles with an origin in statistical process control and the scientific method. In many ways, the methodologies are complementary to each other, and an understanding of both will strengthen improvement work.[2] As improvement work becomes more advanced, an individual or institution may adopt tools from either methodology to best fit their project.

The Model for Improvement

The MFI is a framework for applying the principles of improvement to a QI project. The model comprises three questions: What are we trying to accomplish? How will we know that a change is an improvement? And what changes can we make that will result in an improvement? After asking these questions, small tests of change or Plan-Do-Study-Act (PDSA)[3] cycles help guide the improvement work (Figure 5.1).

We will use the example of an intraoperative handoff process to illustrate how the MFI can guide improvement work. This example will help illustrate the use of SMART aims, PDSAs, and key driver diagrams (KDDs).

A common early improvement project among perioperative teams is improving the handoff process. Consider an anesthesia department that has been getting complaints that handoffs between providers are often incomplete. There was even an adverse event that occurred because the team handing off forgot to mention the presence of a throat pack. The group decides to implement a QI project around intraoperative handoffs.

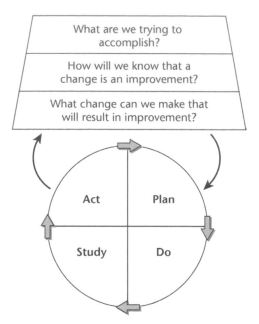

Figure 5.1 Model for Improvement: CCC Rights Link permission obtained 6/10/21

What are we trying to accomplish?

The first question addresses the aim of the improvement project, "What are we trying to accomplish?" An aim should be SMART: Specific, Measurable, Achievable, Relevant, and Timely. Furthermore, the aim of the improvement project should fit into the larger aims of the hospital.

In the above example, the SMART aim was to improve the percent of complete intra-operative handoffs from 60% to 90% in six months. A complete handoff was defined as one that includes all information in a handoff checklist. The team thought a 50% improvement over six months was realistically achievable. They planned to use observers to evaluate the quality of handoffs against a checklist.

How will we know that a change is an improvement?

Asking the second question, "How will we know that a change is an improvement?", requires you to think about what you can measure that will tell you if a change is successful. Choosing measures can be challenging in improvement work, but it is critical to the project.

Three types of measures used in improvement are outcome measures, process measures, and balancing measures. An outcome measure looks at the impact on patients or other stakeholders. A process measure evaluates how the parts or steps in a system are working. Finally, a balancing measure looks at unintended consequences that may result from the change. Which measures are chosen will depend on the specific project. For a simple project, a single outcome or process measure may be adequate; however, sometimes all three measures may be needed.

The intraoperative handoff team used a process measure as their primary measure for the project. The handoff checklist evaluated the quality and reliability of the handoff process. This measure gave them timely feedback to implement interventions and to see the results.

The team also tracked the rate of adverse events that occurred over this time period. An adverse event is an outcome measure. However, adverse events related to handoffs occur infrequently. If this was used as the only measure, it would not give enough feedback for the project.

Some anesthesiologists were concerned that the process would be too cumbersome and would impact their workflow. As a balancing measure, the group decided to make a brief survey measuring anesthesiologists' satisfaction with the handoff process.

What changes can we make that will result in an improvement?

The first step to answer the final question, "What changes can we make that will result in improvement?", is to use current knowledge to brainstorm possible interventions for the project. The interventions are later tested using PDSA cycles. It is helpful to have different stakeholders, or anyone whose role is critical to the process, to get different perspectives. In order to generate ideas for interventions, there are a number of tools that may be of help. Some of these are process maps, failure mode effects analysis (FMEA, discussed in Chapter 10), change concepts, pareto charts, and KDDs. KDDs are described in detail later in this chapter.

The handoff group decided to use a process map and modified FMEA to help them to generate possible interventions. First, the process was outlined from start to finish. Next, everything that could go wrong in each step in the process was listed. Finally, ideas to mitigate each step's potential problems were noted. Some possible interventions were as follows:

1. Requiring both providers to be physically present in the operating room
2. Having a standardized checklist
3. Having the boardrunner (anesthesiologist in charge) notify both attendings

PDSA Cycles

Having brainstormed possible interventions, the next step is to test them. In the MFI, this is done through PDSA, or Plan-Do-Study-Act, cycles. The four steps of a PDSA cycle are described below (Figure 5.2).[3]

1. *Plan*

   The first step is to plan the test and collection of data. When planning, it is often helpful to use who, what, when, where, and why questions. Start small for the first PDSA. In subsequent PDSAs, the scope can be increased. The data at this point is for learning, and it does not have to match the overall measure. It can be objective, such as a measure of time to complete a task, or subjective, such as simply collecting feedback comments.

   The handoff team in our example decided to start small and to test their handoff checklist with three different pairs of providers on a single day. They gave the providers a paper copy of the checklist to use as a guide. A nurse in the room acted as an observer, recording if the handoff took place and if it was complete.

2. *Do*

   Run the test. Collect relevant observations and data. The nurse observer confirmed that the handoffs had taken place but did not always cover all the points in the

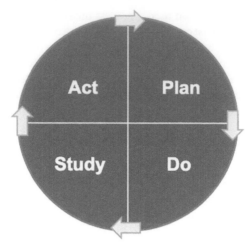

Figure 5.2 Plan-Do-Study-Act: CCC Rights Link permission obtained 6/10/21
(A black and white version of this figure will appear in some formats. For the color version, refer to the plate section.)

checklist. The team asked the anesthesiologists for feedback on how the handoffs went. Overall they liked the checklist. However, they felt that it was disorganized and that the individual points could be arranged in a more logical fashion.

3. *Study*

   How did your results compare to predictions? What new information was learned? The handoff team learned that providers were willing to use the checklist, but that it needed to follow the current workflow.

4. *Act*

   Use what has been learned to plan the next step. Decide to either adopt, adapt, or abandon the test. The handoff team received positive feedback on their checklist with useful suggestions. They decided to *adapt* the checklist by reorganizing it to better match the current workflow before the next PDSA.

With more and more PDSA cycles, knowledge about the project grows. PDSAs may be organized around similar tests, known as PDSA ramps. The handoff team might do a whole ramp of PDSAs on improving the usability of their checklist. PDSAs in this ramp could test the checklist on different days and in different areas, such as MRI or the cath lab. Afterward, another ramp on improving the consistent use of the checklist could be done as a next step. In this ramp, some PDSAs might include testing where to put the paper checklist, combining the checklist with the electronic anesthesia record system, or even educating the department.

Key Driver Diagram

W. Edwards Deming said that information by itself is not knowledge.[1] Information must be combined with a theory to be knowledge. As theories are tested through PDSA cycles, knowledge grows. A KDD is a representation of the current state of knowledge. It is a fluid document. As knowledge increases through testing, the KDD updates to reflect learning.

Example KDD: Intraoperative Handoffs

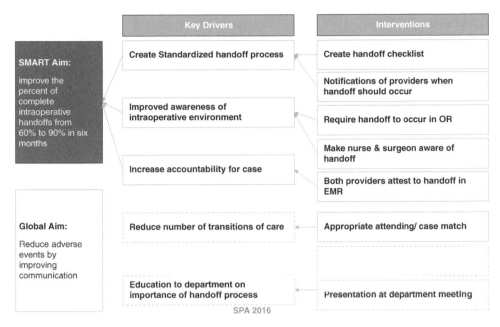

Figure 5.3 Key driver diagram: Permission obtained 6/10/21 IHI
Reprinted from www.IHI.org with permission of the Institute for Healthcare Improvement, ©2021.
(A black and white version of this figure will appear in some formats. For the color version, refer to the plate section.)

A KDD starts by asking what the aim of the project is. The aim should be SMART: Specific, Measurable, Achievable, Relevant, and Timely. Next, the key drivers for the aim are listed. A key driver is anything that will have an impact on the aim. These drivers can be subdivided into primary and secondary drivers. For each key driver, one needs to ask what interventions will target this key driver. Sometimes we think of the key drivers as *what* we are trying to improve, and the interventions as *how* we are trying to improve it. Not all interventions have to be tested at once. Highlighting the interventions and key drivers that are currently being worked on can be a useful way to keep track (Figure 5.3).

The handoff team used the above KDD to keep track of their project. The KDD lists the SMART aim as well as the key drivers and interventions. As more was learned about the handoff process through PDSAs, the KDD was updated.

Lean Approach

The Lean approach strives to engage the "frontline" workers to generate ideas and to enact changes while adding value for the customer, eliminating waste in the production process, and delivering high-quality products. The five key principles are as follows: (1) identify what is valuable to the customer, (2) map the steps to bring product to production in order to identify waste, (3) prioritize steps that impart value, (4) customer's needs dictate what is produced, and (5) consistently improve the system by removing waste. Lean's transition to healthcare began in the 2000s, and the majority of efforts have been focused on operational improvements, as this approach can be especially useful when standardization and efficiency in processes are key goals.[4, 5, 6]

A3 Form

The A3 refers to a single 11 × 17-inch paper that contains a template to guide QI projects[7]. The form is used from top left to bottom right with the left half of the paper used to describe the problem in detail. The first three components of the left half of the A3 include the following: problem statement (be specific), background (why is this problem important to solve?), and current state (target state, actual state, define the gap between). It is important to directly observe current conditions where the work is done in order to define the current state most accurately.

The fourth component of the left side is defining the target statement. As with the MFI methodology, the target statement should be SMART: Specific, Measurable, Achievable, Relevant, and Time-bound. The target statement may change as the root cause analysis progresses and more insight regarding the problem is elucidated.

The last component of the left side of the A3 is the analysis that will allow for the identification of root causes for the problem. It is important to resist the desire to provide interventions and solutions before completing the problem statement and investigation of the root causes. There are a number of tools that can be used to break down the problem and to illustrate the analysis. For example, asking the Five Whys means to continue to ask "why" whenever a problem is encountered in order to discover the root cause. The fishbone diagram as illustrated in the example A3 below is a visual tool to illustrate contributing causes to the problem.

The right side of the A3 is used to demonstrate the proposed countermeasures to the problems identified on the left side. Countermeasures may be organized in the KDD to demonstrate a specific proposed action that directly addresses an existing condition. Alternatively, countermeasures may simply be in list form, each with an owner and time frame, so that progress can be tracked. The countermeasure will create a new situation that may have its own set of problems, so this is a process that will change and evolve in the workplace over time. Countermeasures can be prioritized by the group based on resource allocation and organizational goals. It is also important to include a cost analysis of the proposed new workflow in order to identify hidden costs or savings.

The final piece of the A3 is the sustain plan where owners are assigned to the ongoing activities with clearly defined timelines stated. Plans to reevaluate or to PDCA (Plan-Do-Check-Act) the process can be included in the sustain plan.

There are several other tools in the Lean toolkit, including design events and rapid process improvement workshops, which can be used for bigger projects. Lean uses the concept of 5S (Sort [Seiri], Set in order [Seiton], Shine [Seiso], Standardize [Seiketsu], and Sustain [Shitsuke]) in order to better organize the work space. In every Lean process, the principles of driving out waste, improving flow, and building in quality and safety by standardizing processes are applied.

References

1. Deming WE. *The New Economics for Industry, Government, Education.* 2nd ed., Cambridge, MA, Massachusetts Institute of Technology, Center for Advanced Educational Services, 1994; 106.

2. Best M and Neuhauser D. Heroes & Martyrs of quality and safety: W Edwards Deming: Father of quality management, patient and composer. *Quality & Safety in Health Care.* 2005;14:311.

3. Institute for Healthcare Improvement. QI Essentials Toolkit: PDSA Worksheet. Cambridge, MA, Institute for Healthcare Improvement. Available at ihi.org, www.ihi.org/resources/Pages/Tools/PlanDo StudyActWorksheet.aspx (Accessed 9/6/2020).

4. Afsar-manesh N, Lonowski S, and Namavar AA. Leveraging lean principles in creating a comprehensive quality program: The UCLA health readmission reduction initiative. *Healthcare*. 2017;5(4):194–198.

5. Nathan AT and Kaplan HC. Tools and methods for quality improvement and patient safety in perinatal care. *Seminars in Perinatology*. 2017;41:142.

6. Scoville R and Little K. Comparing lean and quality improvement. *IHI White Paper*. Cambridge, MA, Institute for Healthcare Improvement, 2014; 4,18 (Available at ihi.org).

7. Shool J. *Managing to Learn: Using the A3 Management Process to Solve Problems, Gain Agreement, Mentor, and Lead*. Cambridge, MA, Lean Enterprise Institute, 2008.

6 Cause Analysis

Kristina A. Toncray

Introduction

We all make errors every day. In healthcare, the errors we make can harm our patients. When such an event happens, the institution owes it not only to the patient but also to the staff involved in an event, as well as to future patients who may be similarly harmed, to learn from the event and to prevent similar events from happening again.

There are various types of Cause Analysis, or tools used to analyze the causes of certain events. Usually such tools are used to study an undesired outcome, and in healthcare, these are often used to study adverse events. This chapter will describe the process of performing a Root Cause Analysis (RCA) for serious events, as well as touch upon the concepts of Apparent Cause Analysis for less serious events and Common Cause Analysis to look for themes across events. Failure Mode Effects Analysis (FMEA), related to Cause Analysis, is described separately in Chapter 10.

Nomenclature and Terminology

"Adverse events" are adverse occurrences associated with medical care and may result from error (e.g., medication errors or diagnostic errors) or may be an adverse reaction or negative outcome of treatment.[1] They are often, but not always, preventable and thus are not synonymous with medical error events or with preventable events. The type of review required for different adverse events will be determined by your institution's event classification system.

"Sentinel events" are those events that cause serious injury (e.g., death or "loss of limb or function") that are listed among the National Quality Forum's (NQF) list of serious reportable events, originally created in 2002. The term, though widely used to mean "serious adverse event" by those who use it, specifically refers to those events that should be reported to various reporting bodies. The Joint Commission, for example, uses this term when describing events that should be reported to them. This list includes certain types of adverse events but is not a complete list of all the safety events that can occur within healthcare settings. Adverse events, safety events, harm events, or preventable harm events are not necessarily synonymous with the concept of "sentinel events," so this term should only be used when referring specifically to the NQF list.[1, 2]

A Brief History of Cause Analysis in Healthcare

The tools and terms for investigating and analyzing cases arose from the engineering concepts of "failure analysis" or "failure investigation." RCA is the most well known of these concepts, and though it was originally developed to study industrial accidents, it has, in the last few decades, become a standard and fairly widespread tool within healthcare to study undesired, usually preventable patient outcomes.

Many healthcare institutions have modeled their original systems after the Veterans' Affairs Administration's RCA structure or the Joint Commission's "Framework for Conducting a Root Cause Analysis and Action Plan" that provides templated steps for conducting an RCA. This template addresses issues such as intended process flow, missed steps in the process, human factors, equipment issues, communication, staffing, competencies, culture, and other areas in the organization that could experience a similar failure, then requires planned actions for each identified finding.[3] The Joint Commission has required an RCA for review of sentinel events since 1997, and many states require the same.[4]

Root Cause Analysis

RCA is a structured tool used rigorously to study a case, usually a serious adverse event; it analyzes the errors that lead to an undesired outcome and supports creation of action items to prevent the case from occurring again. It is a classic example of a tool that uses a systems approach, rather than an individual approach, of error analysis,[4] though experts recommend that individual errors cannot be ignored during the analysis and must be well understood to keep similar individual errors from recurring. The goal of an RCA is to find out what happened, why it happened, and how to prevent it from happening again.[5]

Ideally, an RCA takes place fairly soon after an event has occurred. Waiting too long after an event has happened is not ideal as other issues or events can start to take priority over the one in question.

It is important to note that, by definition, a RCA is a retrospective analysis tool. It does allow healthcare organizations to identify threats to safety that may cause future harm, but only after an event has already happened; thus, prospective analysis methods such as simulation (discussed in Chapter 2) and FMEA (discussed in Chapter 10) should be used when the goal is to prevent an adverse event from ever happening.

What is a "Root Cause"?

A root cause is the most fundamental reason why an event occurred.[1] Each root cause identified during a RCA should have an action item in the final action plan that will prevent or mitigate an undesirable outcome in the future.[3]

RCAs will likely also uncover "contributing factors," or additional reasons that are not necessarily the root or most basic reasons, that led to the event.[1]

Guiding Principles

An RCA, including action items generated, focuses on systems causes, rather than on individual blame. Individual error is not ignored but rather used as a starting point to analyze why that error occurred and how it led to patient harm. Thus, it is part of an effort to move beyond a culture of blame and toward a robust culture of safety within healthcare institutions. RCAs should be as impartial as possible and should focus on prevention, not punishment.[5]

RCA relies on the team digging deeply "at each level of cause and effect" in order to find the true, deep, root causes of problems in healthcare.[5] Often this is done via the "5

Whys,"[6, 7] a technique attributed to Taichi Ohno of Toyota and used throughout production, healthcare, and other industries to get to a deep understanding of a problem. The human body and the healthcare system are complex, so events that lead to patient harm within healthcare systems are therefore often complex as well. Adverse events usually occur via an alignment of multiple factors. By asking "why" over and over again, one ensures that the simple answer (often "human error") is not accepted, and that the solution will truly fix, rather than mask, the problems.

Choosing Cases for RCA

RCA is typically done when something needs to be studied in depth. The goal is to put systems in place that would prevent a similar outcome from occurring in the future. Various institutions have different ways to classify events and thus different thresholds for types of cases they review in RCA. Some institutions only conduct RCA for cases in which there was significant harm to a patient. Other institutions also conduct RCAs for "close call" or "near miss" events, or those in which harm to the patient was avoided based on chance or timely intervention; these occur much more frequently in healthcare than do harmful events and are a tremendous opportunity for learning prior to actual patient harm.[1, 5] We recommend using a risk-based classification system in order to apply some rigor to case selection. There are various classification systems in use across various hospital systems. One example from the VA is their "Safety Assessment Code," or SAC, based on the severity of an incident (including extent of impairment, length of stay, and level of care required to treat the injury) and the probability of recurrence.

Note that "intentional unsafe acts" are not appropriate for analysis via RCA. These are events that result from purposely unsafe acts, including those that are criminal or related to substance abuse by a provider.[1]

Members of an RCA Team

An RCA should have, ideally, no more than four to six people on the team in order to maximize the team's ability to be productive. The team should be composed of people from various disciplines, and there should be people both familiar and unfamiliar with the process being studied.[8] Leaders of an organization must also be included in the RCA process in order to remove barriers to change.[5]

At some institutions, those directly involved in an event are on an RCA team. Other systems specifically do not include those involved in an event in the meeting. The newest recommendations from the National Patient Safety Foundation endorse not including those involved in an event at the review. The review team must talk openly about the event and may refrain from speaking their complete thoughts if someone involved in the event is present, in order to spare their feelings. At Seattle Children's Hospital, we have also found this to be the case and do not invite those involved in an event but rather interview them prior to the review so that we have their perspective and opinions.

Finally, one should consider the inclusion of a patient or family representative. At Seattle Children's Hospital, standard practice is to invite an RCA-trained member of the Family Advisory Council to event reviews to represent the patient and parent perspective.

Steps in a RCA

1. Determine if an RCA is the appropriate tool for a particular case: see section on *"choosing cases for RCA."*
2. Choose a team: see section on *"members of an RCA team."*
3. Collect information (both facts and people's perspectives) in order to "reconstruct the event."[4] This is often done via chart review, interviews, and process walks.
4. Map out the process: what happened in the case in question, what usually happens and what should ideally happen.
5. Identify what happened: what errors or missed opportunities contributed to the undesired outcome? A proper RCA identifies these based on accurate information, including the medical record and interviews of those involved. Assumptions have no place within an RCA.
6. Analyze the case: what are the causes of the event? Some are direct causes, while some may be contributing factors that only indirectly led to the event. The team should identify both how and why the event occurred (identification of active errors by individuals as well as identification and analysis of latent errors engrained in the system).[4]
7. "Ask why five times" in order to identify the true root cause(s).[6, 7]
8. Write causal statements, or statements that link the identified causes above to the effects (the undesired outcome in question). Causal statements should generally meet the following five rules:[1]
   a. Causal statements must clearly show the "cause and effect" relationship.
   b. Negative descriptors (e.g., poorly, inadequate) are not used in causal statements.
   c. Each human error must have a preceding cause.
   d. Each procedural deviation must have a preceding cause.
   e. Failure to act is only causal when there was a preexisting duty to act.
9. Create an action plan consisting of action items that will prevent the error from happening again in the future. Actions are broken down into strong, intermediate, and weak actions per the National Center for Patient Safety (NCPS).[5]
   The action plan should address system and process deficiencies identified during the RCA, and outcome measures that prove that the deficiencies are "effectively eliminated, controlled, or accepted."[1] In the spirit of quality improvement, actions should ideally be tested in a small area prior to full implementation.
10. Write, disseminate, and review "Lessons Learned" from the event.[8] (Table 6.1).[5]

Table 6.1 Action items from RCA[5]

	Strong	Intermediate	Weak
Definition	Likely to eliminate or greatly reduce the likelihood of an event	Likely to control the root cause or vulnerability	By itself less likely to be effective
Examples	Physical plant changes, forcing functions that prevent common mistakes	Standardization of equipment, simplification of a process, cognitive aids (checklists, labels, mnemonics), redundancy (backups, double checks)	Education, policy change

Tools Typically Used in the RCA Process

Process Map

The Process Map is a visual description of a process, often describing not just what happened in a particular case but also what usually happens or what is supposed to happen (Figure 6.1).

Cause and effect diagram

The cause and effect diagram, often called a fishbone or Ishikawa diagram, is a visual representation of all the possible causes of a certain effect. On the right of the visual, the outcome in question is labeled. On the left-hand side of the diagram, the group lists all the possible contributing factors to that outcome, grouped into various categories (Figure 6.2).

The Institute for Healthcare Improvement (IHI) proposes a number of different categories, such as patient characteristics, task factors, individual staff members, team factors, work environment, organizational and management factors, and institutional context. Other groups have proposed other categories, such as communication, training, fatigue, scheduling, equipment, policies, and procedures.[1] The user should feel free to use the categories that work best for the event in question. Below are examples of the types of errors that fall into the various categories above (Table 6.2).

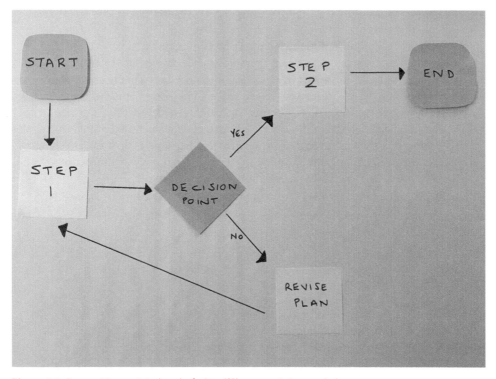

Figure 6.1 Process Map – original work of editor (SR), no permission needed
(A black and white version of this figure will appear in some formats. For the color version, refer to the plate section.)

FISHBONE DIAGRAM

PROBLEM **CAUSES**

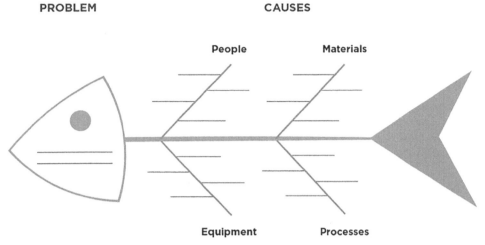

Figure 6.2 Fishbone – From SCH toolbox, no SCH logo, no permission needed
(A black and white version of this figure will appear in some formats. For the color version, refer to the plate section.)

Table 6.2 Factors that may lead to latent errors

Type of Factor	Example
Institutional/regulatory	A patient on anticoagulants received an intramuscular pneumococcal vaccination, resulting in a hematoma and prolonged hospitalization. The hospital was under regulatory pressure to improve its pneumococcal vaccination rates.
Organizational/management	A nurse detected a medication error, but the physician discouraged the nurse from reporting it.
Work environment	Lacking the appropriate equipment to perform hysteroscopy, operating room staff improvised using equipment from other sets. During the procedure, the patient suffered an air embolism.
Team environment	A surgeon completed an operation despite being informed by a nurse and the anesthesiologist that the suction catheter tip was missing. The tip was subsequently found inside the patient, requiring reoperation.
Staffing	An overworked nurse mistakenly administered insulin instead of an antiemetic medication, resulting in hypoglycemic coma.
Task-related	An intern incorrectly calculated the equivalent dose of long-acting MS Contin for a patient who had been receiving Vicodin. The patient experienced an opiate overdose and aspiration pneumonia, resulting in a prolonged ICU course.
Patient characteristics	The parents of a young child misread the instructions on a bottle of acetaminophen, causing their child to experience liver damage.

Action plan

The action plan lists what actions are already in place or are going to be enacted in order to prevent the errors that allowed the event in question to occur. Action plans should be specific and include an owner of the action item, an implementation date, and an associated measure of effectiveness. Note that a measure of effectiveness is different from a measure of completion and should ideally be a process or outcome measure that indicates that the item is in fact preventing the errors in question.

Root Cause Analysis[2]

Based on nationwide inconsistencies in the success of learning from RCA, the National Patient Safety Foundation convened a panel of national experts and stakeholders and issued the "Root Cause Analysis and Action (RCA[2])" best practice guidelines in order to standardize and improve the RCA process.[8] The goal of this new suggested process is to focus effort on the implementation of sustainable action items: "The most important step in the RCA[2] process is the identification and implementation of actions to eliminate or control system hazards or vulnerabilities that have been identified in the contributing factor statements."[4] For example, the guidelines explicitly state that at least one intermediate or strong action item should be identified in each action plan. The recommendations emphasize accountability, in the form of individual ownership of action items (over committees), and the need for active leadership involvement and oversight. Other recommendations include timing standards (convening a review within 72 hours of recognition), prioritization of RCA[2] work for those on an analysis team, and the need for closed-loop communication to those involved in an event. They also encourage interviewing patients and families after an event.

Apparent Cause Analysis

Apparent Cause Analysis is a tool that can be used for less serious events or when one does not have the time or resources to devote to a full RCA. Apparent Cause Analysis requires the user to describe the event, define the problem and its significance and consequences, address errors and equipment issues, describe the apparent cause of the event, create and explain appropriate corrective actions, and identify trends. Though some people tend to use the phrases "Root Cause Analysis" and "Apparent Cause Analysis" interchangeably, an Apparent Cause Analysis should not take as much time as a full RCA as, by definition, it only studies the obvious causes, rather than the deeper ones that may take some digging and require asking "why" five times.

In their paper describing their use of Apparent Cause Analysis to study Healthcare-Associated Infections (HAIs) in their Pediatric Intensive Care Units, Bogue et al.[9] described their need to study central line associated bloodstream infections (CLABSIs) via Apparent Cause Analysis in order to understand the events, prior to analyzing the events in aggregate. A standard ACA template is used for all CLABSIs, which includes information such as patient name, unit, organism, labs, and other details (e.g., chlorhexidine bathing, oral hygiene, line complications, number of flushes, and lab draws) in order to look for errors. Information is then entered into a database following each investigation for aggregate analysis.

Common Cause Analysis

Often called "Common Cause Failure Analysis" and sometimes "Systemic Cause Analysis," Common Cause Analysis originated in the engineering world and looks at multiple events in aggregate in order to study themes from individual case analyses.

Bogue et al.[9] described this type of aggregate analysis, which they used to study HAIs in aggregate to find trends and to search for new mitigation and infection prevention strategies. The advantages of this type of analysis were made clear in one unit that was seeing a significant spike in CLABSIs. ACAs had identified possible causes such as issues with hand hygiene, but only when a Systemic Cause Analysis was completed did the unit learn that the spike in infections appeared due to use of a new blood draw system. Removal of the new device brought the CLABSI rate back down to the previous baseline. Only aggregate analysis was able to identify the cause of this infection rate increase, which had not been noted during previous individual case analyses.

Mallet et al.[10] published their Common Cause Analysis of eight wrong site, procedure or patient events that occurred over a two-year period. Each of the events were studied initially via traditional RCA. Then all eight cases were studied in aggregate to look for trends. The goal was to determine overall common causes of these events. The authors found that, of 59 errors across all cases, after sorting by NCPS Triage Card categories,[11] 22 errors were in the area of "Rules, Policies, and Procedures." Seventeen errors were in the category of "Scheduling and Fatigue." They focused their efforts on reducing wrong site, procedure or patient events to these top two categories. Since those efforts, they have not had further such adverse events in the year prior to publication. This type of analysis allowed them to prioritize their efforts rather than waste effort on themes that may have been isolated to one or two cases, or to work on action items for individual cases in isolation rather than integrating efforts. RCA and common cause analysis are compared in Table 6.3.[11]

Crea and Clapper[12] describe the use of Common Cause Analysis to study medication errors in a large hospital system. Event reviewers collected standard data for each case identified by a trigger tool, which was then collated and analyzed. Over a three-year period, the overall reduction in adverse events had decreased by 50% following implementation of action items to address the highest priority common causes.[12]

Finally, the Children's Hospital of Philadelphia uses Common Cause Analysis on an annual basis in order to prioritize issues for hospital executive leadership.[11] By sorting errors and concepts from approximately 25 of the most serious events into various headings (also via NCPS Triage Card categories, as above) and scoring, similar to an FMEA, for severity, occurrence, and detection, they are able to assign Risk Priority Numbers (RPNs) to the themes. Causes and themes with RPNs of more than 250 (usually five to six per year) are shared in the report, so the institution is able to incorporate the most important issues into the institutional operating plan for the next fiscal year as prioritized patient safety and quality goals.

Aggregate RCA

Slightly different in concept from Common Cause Analysis, in which separate analyses are conducted prior to looking at learnings from multiple cases, Aggregate RCA is used to study a group of near miss or close call cases.[8] Topics studied via this review tool are

Table 6.3 Comparison of root cause analysis and common cause analysis

Root Cause Analysis	Common Cause Analysis
Single case or a few related cases.	Many or all cases.
Event directed (examines a single event or adverse trend of related events).	Time or trend directed (examines all cases in a time period).
Efficient for diagnosing process, protocol, and technology causes.	Efficient for diagnosing people, leadership, and environment of care causes.
Investigates cause-and-effect relationships directly.	Infers cause-and-effect relationships using existing analyses.
An effective program lowers rates of serious harm by 50% every two years.	An effective program lowers rates of serious patient harm by 50% every two years, with 10% the resource allocation of root cause analysis.

usually high-risk, high-volume cases, predetermined at an institution, such as patient falls and medication errors, and trends are identified across similar events to support focus areas for improvement.[13]

Conclusion

There are various methods available to study adverse events in healthcare. The tools above provide some rigor and structure to the investigation of undesired events and the prevention of future similar events. Though these tools can be time- and resource-intensive, the imperative for those who work in healthcare quality and patient safety is continually to improve upon current processes by studying undesired events and preventing future patient harm.

References

1. U.S. Department of Veterans Affairs. VA National Center for Patient Safety, Glossary of Patient Safety Terms; 2015. Available at www.patientsafety.va.gov/professionals/publications/glossary.asp (Accessed 5/6/21).

2. The National Quality Forum. Serious Reportable Events; 2009. Available at www.qualityforum.org/Topics/SREs/Serious_Reportable_Events.aspx (Accessed 9/13/2020).

3. The Joint Commission. Patient Safety Topics, Sentinel Event. The RCA2: Improving Root Cause Analyses and Actions to Prevent Harm; 2015. Available at www.jointcommission.org/-/media/tjc/documents/resources/patient-safety-topics/sentinel-event/rca_framework_101017.pdf?db=web&hash=B2B439317A20C3D1982F9FBB94E1724B (Accessed 9/13/2020).

4. Agency for Healthcare Research and Quality. Patient Safety Primer, Root Cause Analysis; 2019. Available at https://psnet.ahrq.gov/primers/primer/10/root-cause-analysis (Accessed 9/13/2020).

5. U.S. Department of Veterans Affairs. VA National Center for Patient Safety, Root Cause Analysis; 2018. Available at www.patientsafety.va.gov/professionals/onthejob/rca.asp (Accessed 9/13/2020).

6. Toyota Motor Asia Pacific. Ask "Why" Five Times about Every Matter; 2014–2016. Available at www.toyota-myanmar.com/about-toyota/toyota-traditions/quality/ask-why-five-times-about-every-matter#:~:text=%E2%80%9CAsk%20'why'%20five%20times,Why%20did%20the%20robot%20stop%3F%E2%80%9D (Accessed 9/13/2020).

7. Institute for Healthcare Improvement. Ask "Why" Five Times to Get to the Root Cause; 2020. Available at www.ihi.org/resources/Pages/ImprovementStories/AskWhyFiveTimestoGettotheRootCause.aspx/ (Accessed 9/13/2020).

8. Institute for Healthcare Improvement. RCA2: Improving Root Cause Analyses and Actions to Prevent Harm; 2016. Available at www.ihi.org/resources/Pages/Tools/RCA2-Improving-Root-Cause-Analyses-and-Actions-to-Prevent-Harm.aspx (Accessed 7/10/2022).

9. Bogue TL and Bogue RL. Unbundling the bundles: Using apparent and systemic cause analysis to prevent health care-associated infection in pediatric intensive care units. *Critical Care Nursing Clinics of North America.* 2017;29(2):217–231.

10. Mallett R, Conroy M, Saslaw LZ, et al. Preventing wrong site, procedure, and patient events using a common cause analysis. *American Journal of Medical Quality.* 2012;27:21–29.

11. Browne AM, Mullen R, Teets J, et al. Common cause analysis: Focus on institutional change. *Advances in Patient Safety: New Directions and Alternative Approaches* (Vol. 1: Assessment). Henriksen K, Battles JB, Keyes MA, et al., eds., Rockville, MD, Agency for Healthcare Research and Quality; August 2008. Table 1, Department of Veterans Affairs National Center for Patient Safety triage categories. Available from: www.ncbi.nlm.nih.gov/books/NBK43639/table/advances-browne_5.t1/

12. Clapper C, Crea K. Common Cause Analysis. Patient Safety & Quality Healthcare; 2010. Available at www.psqh.com/analysis/common-cause-analysis/ (Accessed 9/13/2020).

13. Neily J, et al. Using aggregate root cause analysis to improve patient safety. *The Joint Commission Journal on Quality and Safety.* 2003;29(8):434–439.

Reporting Adverse Events

Rebecca Claure and Julianne Mendoza

Adverse Event Reporting

Identification of medical errors and adverse events is necessary to understand the current safety environment and the opportunities to minimize harm and to improve safety. A major barrier to progress in quality improvement and safety has been the inability to identify and measure these events with accuracy and consistency.[1, 2, 3] Many different methods and sources of data have been utilized to identify and measure medical errors and adverse events with varying degrees of success. The types of events and the frequency of events detected can be variable and will depend on the method and the source of data used to measure these events.[1, 4, 5]

The Institute of Medicine defines a medical error as "the failure to complete a planned action as intended or the use of a wrong plan to achieve an aim."[6] Adverse events are injuries that result from medical interventions rather than the underlying disease or condition of the patient.[6, 7] It is important to differentiate between medical errors that do not lead to patient harm and errors that result in adverse events and actual patient harm.[2] Public health research has confirmed that only 10%–20% of errors are reported and that the vast majority of these reported errors cause no harm to patients.[8] Of errors that cause adverse events, the majority are preventable.[9, 10, 11]

The main purpose of any of the following measurement methods is the potential for learning from the individual circumstances that led to the actual adverse event or potential adverse event (near miss). By identifying these events, reviewing the apparent causes and underlying factors, and then using that knowledge to implement system fixes to prevent similar events in the future, the risk of future patient harm is minimized.[12]

Methods used to measure medical errors will be detailed in this chapter and include provider reported events, retrospective chart reviews, trigger tools, national clinical registries, administrative data, and patient or family reported events. Analysis of adverse events was covered in Chapter 6.

Provider Reported Events

Event reporting by providers has a long history. Initially, these reports were often anecdotal and communicated to colleagues by word of mouth. Anesthesiologists soon began to focus on the most catastrophic "incidents" associated with anesthesia.[13] The technique of critical incident analysis was first introduced by Flanagan in 1954.[14] Critical incident monitoring is most commonly associated with the aviation industry but is also used in other high-risk industries. Anesthesiology was the first medical specialty to adopt incident reporting as a safety tool.[15, 16] Critical incident reporting is now well established in both anesthesiology and critical care, as well as in other medical and surgical specialties.

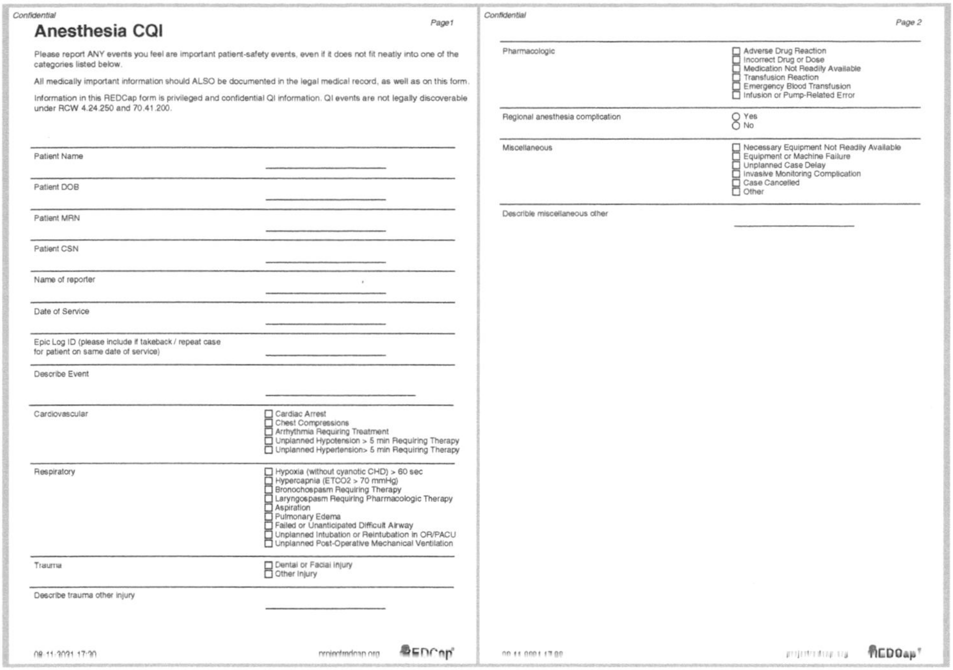

Confidential

Page1

Anesthesia CQI

Please report ANY events you feel are important patient-safety events, even if it does not fit neatly into one of the categories listed below.

All medically important information should ALSO be documented in the legal medical record, as well as on this form.

Information in this REDCap form is privileged and confidential QI information. QI events are not legally discoverable under RCW 4.24.250 and 70.41.200.

Patient Name

Patient DOB

Patient MRN

Patient CSN

Name of reporter

Date of Service

Epic Log ID (please include if takeback / repeat case for patient on same date of service)

Describe Event

Cardiovascular
- ☐ Cardiac Arrest
- ☐ Chest Compressions
- ☐ Arrhythmia Requiring Treatment
- ☐ Unplanned Hypotension > 5 min Requiring Therapy
- ☐ Unplanned Hypertension> 5 min Requiring Therapy

Respiratory
- ☐ Hypoxia (without cyanotic CHD) > 60 sec
- ☐ Hypercapnia (ETCO2 > 70 mmHg)
- ☐ Bronchospasm Requiring Therapy
- ☐ Laryngospasm Requiring Pharmacologic Therapy
- ☐ Aspiration
- ☐ Pulmonary Edema
- ☐ Failed or Unanticipated Difficult Airway
- ☐ Unplanned Intubation or Reintubation in OR/PACU
- ☐ Unplanned Post-Operative Mechanical Ventilation

Trauma
- ☐ Dental or Facial Injury
- ☐ Other Injury

Describe trauma other injury

REDCap

Confidential

Page 2

Pharmacologic
- ☐ Adverse Drug Reaction
- ☐ Incorrect Drug or Dose
- ☐ Medication Not Readily Available
- ☐ Transfusion Reaction
- ☐ Emergency Blood Transfusion
- ☐ Infusion or Pump-Related Error

Regional anesthesia complication
- ○ Yes
- ○ No

Miscellaneous
- ☐ Necessary Equipment Not Readily Available
- ☐ Equipment or Machine Failure
- ☐ Unplanned Case Delay
- ☐ Invasive Monitoring Complication
- ☐ Case Cancelled
- ☐ Other

Describle miscellaneous other

REDCap

Figure 7.1 Reporting template – Anesthesia CQI blank from SCH, which did not require permission for its use (A black and white version of this figure will appear in some formats. For the color version, refer to the plate section.)

Voluntary incident reporting by providers is one of the most widely used methods to measure both errors and adverse events associated with medical care.[17, 18, 19] These reports allow for review and analysis of the identified events so that improvement opportunities are recognized, interventions to mitigate the identified opportunities can be developed, and these interventions can be evaluated for efficacy.[1, 20] Systematic capture and analysis of these reports allows data about incidence and potential risk to be acquired.[1, 20] The greater the number of events reported, the more likely rare events will be captured.[13] Many anesthesiology departmental programs and professional societies depend on voluntary incident reporting systems to guide their quality assurance and quality improvement programs.[12, 16, 21] An example of an electronic anesthesia incident reporting template is shown in Figure 7.1.

Events identified by departmental incident reporting systems can be analyzed in either the appropriate peer review structure or in a departmental quality improvement committee to identify the opportunities for improvement and to design the subsequent system changes.

Voluntary reporting of adverse events and near misses requires engagement of all healthcare providers, including physicians. A reluctance to report events is common among physicians,[13, 16, 18] and physicians as a group utilize voluntary incident reporting systems at a lower rate than other professional groups within healthcare.[13, 16, 22]

In a recent survey of anesthesia providers at an academic institution, barriers to reporting events included an uncertainty of when an incident met criteria for reporting, variability in each individual's threshold for reporting, no perceived benefit to either the patient or the reporter, lack of feedback to the reporter, and fear of professional repercussions.[16] Other disincentives to reporting adverse events include lack of anonymity, concern over confidentiality, shame, fear of implicating others, absence of a supportive forum for disclosure, lack of time, and reporting systems that are complicated or poorly designed.[13, 23, 24]

Learning from incidents and the desire to transform incidents into safety improvements are powerful motivators to reporting events.[16] Other factors that motivate reporting include a system that is accessible and easy to use, data that are captured in a secure and nondiscoverable format, and feedback to reporters.[13, 16, 25] Allowing for anonymous reporting of adverse events, as seen in some hospital-based incident reporting systems, may increase reporting by negating the fear of consequences or distrust of the system.[13, 25] Addressing identified barriers and supporting motivators to reporting can lead to a sustained increase in reporting rates among physicians.[16]

Clinical factors have also been found to impact reporting rates. Factors associated with greater use of a reporting system include increased complexity of procedure, longer duration of surgery, seniority of trainees, and the presence of anesthesia-related complications with the potentially higher risk of litigation.[18] Factors associated with less use of a reporting system include emergency procedures and procedures in which there was no anesthesia trainee involved.[18] Many staff do not consider near misses to be reportable incidents.

Several institutions have demonstrated the efficacy of adopting a force function to mandate quality assurance documentation before closing the electronic medical record (EMR).[16, 19] Mandatory incident reporting systems integrated in the anesthesia information management system have multiple benefits, including capturing every anesthetic performed to determine incident rates and allowing for secure and legally protected data entry that is integrated into the providers' workflow for ease of data entry.[16]

The strengths of voluntary incident reporting include data that is easy to collect, provider-driven reporting that engages frontline personnel, and the opportunity to collect data on near misses. The limitations of relying on providers to report include underreporting of events and a selection bias in events reported. When an adverse event is underreported, the incidence rate of that specific event will be inaccurately low. Interventions to address limitations of self-reporting range from culture change to force functions embedded in the EMR.[16]

Retrospective Chart Review

Retrospective chart review has been considered the gold standard for identifying adverse events since it involves a comprehensive and detailed review of the patient's medical record by healthcare professionals.[26] Retrospective chart review as employed in the Harvard Medical Practice Study (HMPS) is a standard methodology used in a number of international studies to determine adverse event rates.[1, 27] In the HMPS, nurses and medical records administrators trained in the study methods first applied the screening criteria to all the randomly selected patient records. Then, if a record met one or more of the criteria, it was referred for physician review by two independent physician reviewers.[27, 28]

There are multiple limitations to relying on retrospective chart reviews. Reviews of the chart are both labor- and time-intensive, and the review is limited to the information available in the chart, which can be incomplete and of variable quality.[2, 28] Consistency between reviewers is a potential issue for any chart review study, and standardized training of reviewers has been recommended as a way to increase inter-rater reliability and decrease screening errors.[29] Adverse events discovered after discharge are likely to remain undetected unless they result in a readmission. Retrospective chart review remains an impractical method for routine adverse event detection.

Trigger Tool Methodology

Trigger tools were developed to more accurately identify, quantify, and track adverse events causing patient harm.[2, 8, 30] The concept of a "trigger" to identify adverse events in the medical record was introduced by Jick in 1974.[9] One of the benefits of the trigger tool methodology is that adverse event detection is independent of voluntary reporting by healthcare providers. The theory behind trigger tools is that some errors in care will cause a response that can be "tracked."[5, 8, 30]

Discrete data points such as a specific medication or specific lab or vital sign value are most easily utilized for trigger tool reports. Classen developed an automated system to allow detection of adverse drug events (ADEs) using the electronic hospital information system.[31] Automated detection of potential ADEs relied on "triggers" such as sudden medication stop orders, "corrective" medication orders, and selected abnormal lab values.[31] These markers, or triggers, then serve to initiate a more detailed chart review to determine whether an adverse event occurred.[2, 3, 31] For example, a patient who received too much narcotic might require treatment with an opiate antagonist such as naloxone. Naloxone use serves as the trigger to prompt further review to determine whether an adverse event occurred.

The Global Trigger Tool (GTT) was developed in 2003 by the Institute for Healthcare Improvement (IHI) as an easy to use, less labor-intensive method of accurately identifying adverse events and measuring the rate of adverse events over time, alternative to a detailed retrospective chart review.[1, 8, 30] The GTT uses trigger tool methodology and applies it in a more comprehensive way to systematically identify adverse events and harm in adult inpatients.[8] The GTT uses a larger list of triggers (50+) than the HMPS retrospective chart review methodology. By using a broader definition of adverse events and a larger number of triggers, the GTT has identified higher rates of adverse events (20%–30%) than were previously identified by other methodologies (Figure 7.2).[1, 32]

The IHI GTT is organized in modules including medical care (transfusion or use of blood products, resuscitation events, etc.), surgical care (return to surgery or change in procedure, admission to intensive care), and a medication module (flumazenil or naloxone administration).[8] A comprehensive list of the GTT triggers is shown in Table 1. Several different trigger tools are available for use in a variety of healthcare settings such as general care units, intensive care units, ambulatory settings, and for review of medication management.[2, 8] Stockwell et al. have developed a pediatric trigger tool to allow adverse event detection in pediatric inpatient settings.[3]

Trigger tool methodology relies on a manual retrospective review of a random sample of inpatient hospital records using the chosen trigger tool.[2, 8] Since the review relies on sampling to find adverse events, it is critical to use a truly random process for selecting the patient records[8] so that the events identified are truly representative of care at that particular healthcare institution. If using the GTT, two primary reviewers (usually experienced RNs) review the chart independently to look for the presence of triggers.[8] When a "positive" trigger is identified, the record is further reviewed to determine whether an adverse event occurred. Not all positive triggers will correlate with an adverse event.[1, 2, 8] For example, the finding that an X-ray was taken during the procedure is a positive trigger and could indicate that an adverse event occurred but could also be part of standard hospital procedure such as a routine X-ray taken for verification of central line placement. Once the primary reviewers have reached a consensus, a physician reviewer assesses the findings with the primary reviewers to reach a final agreement on the type, number, and severity of events.[1, 8]

Cares Module Triggers	+	Event Description and Harm Category (E-I)	Medication Module Triggers	+	Event Description and Harm Category (E-I)
C1 Transfusion or use of blood products			M1 Clostridium difficile positive stool		
C2 Code/arrest/rapid response team			M2 Partial thromboplastin time greater than 100 seconds		
C3 Acute dialysis					
C4 Positive blood culture			M3 International Normalized Ratio (INR) greater than 6		
C5 X-ray or Doppler studies for emboli or DVT					
C6 Decrease of greater than 25% in hemoglobin or hematocrit			M4 Glucose less than 50 mg/dl		
			M5 Rising BUN or serum creatinine greater than 2 times baseline		
C7 Patient fall					
C8 Pressure ulcers			M6 Vitamin K administration		
C9 Readmission within 30 days			M7 Benadryl (Diphenhydramine) use		
C10 Restraint use			M8 Romazicon (Flumazenil) use		
C11 Healthcare-associated infection			M9 Naloxone (Narcan) use		
C12 In-hospital stroke			M10 Anti-emetic use		
C13 Transfer to higher level of care			M11 Over-sedation/hypotension		
C14 Any procedure complication			M12 Abrupt medication stop		
C15 Other			M13 Other		
Surgical Module Triggers			**Intensive Care Module Triggers**		
S1 Return to surgery			I1 Pneumonia onset		
S2 Change in procedure			I2 Readmission to intensive care		
S3 Admission to intensive care post-op			I3 In-unit procedure		
S4 Intubation/reintubation/BiPap in Post Anesthesia Care Unit (PACU)			I4 Intubation/reintubation		
S5 X-ray intra-op or in PACU			**Perinatal Module Triggers**		
S6 Intra-op or post-op death			P1 Terbutaline use		
S7 Mechanical ventilation greater than 24 hours post-op			P2 3rd- or 4th-degree lacerations		
			P3 Platelet count less than 50,000		
S8 Intra-op epinephrine, norepinephrine, naloxone, or romazicon			P4 Estimated blood loss > 500 ml (vaginal) or > 1,000 ml (C-section)		
S9 Post-op troponin level greater than 1.5 ng/ml			P5 Specialty consult		
			P6 Oxytocic agents		
S10 Injury, repair, or removal of organ			P7 Instrumented delivery		
S11 Any operative complication			P8 General anesthesia		
			Emergency Department Module Triggers		
			E1 Readmission to ED within 48 hours		
			E2 Time in ED greater than 6 hours		

Patient Identifer _____ Total Events_____ Total LOS _____ Write descriptions of the events in greater detail on reverse of Worksheet.

[Photocopy Worksheet single-sided. Leave opposite side blank for notes.]

Figure 7.2 IHI Global Trigger Tool. Reproduced with permission from IHI

Though trigger tool methodology is meant to identify a predetermined trigger rather than to identify an actual adverse event, it has been found to be a reliable and consistent method of detecting adverse events and patient harm.[2, 32, 33] Trigger tools provide a systematic methodology to provide adverse event data through a random sampling approach that allows healthcare systems to determine adverse event rates and understand the areas where quality improvement is necessary. Other advantages to trigger tool methodology are that the technique is flexible and can be customized for use in all clinical environments to allow detection of multiple types of adverse events.[2, 3, 8] Adverse events causing patient harm are identified more frequently with trigger tool use than by voluntary reporting.[32, 34] Rutberg et al. reported that only 6.3% of the adverse events detected by the GTT were reported by staff.[34] Classen et al. reported that the GTT found at least 10 times more adverse events as voluntary reporting.[32] However, voluntary reporting can provide information on near miss events not detected by trigger tool methodology.[3, 35]

National Clinical Registries

Clinical registries (also discussed in Chapter 9) are structured data collection systems that gather uniform data to evaluate specified outcomes for a population defined by a particular disease, condition, or exposure and that serve one or more scientific, clinical, or policy purposes.[36] There are several successful surgical society clinical registries that were established to collect data to facilitate improving surgical quality and patient safety, including the American College of Surgeons National Surgical Quality Improvement Program (NSQIP) and the Society of Thoracic Surgeons (STS) national registry. The STS national registry has several components, including databases focused on general thoracic surgery, adult cardiac surgery, and congenital cardiac surgery. Studies have shown that overall surgical quality has improved in hospitals participating in NSQIP.[37, 38, 39, 40]

The Anesthesia Quality Institute (AQI) was established by the American Society of Anesthesiologists (ASA)in 2008 with the vision to advance the quality and safety of anesthesia care in the United States through aggregation and reporting of clinical and administrative data.[41, 42] The AQI maintains multiple data registries that focus on different aspects of anesthesia practice, including the National Anesthesia Clinical Outcomes Registry (NACOR), the Anesthesia Incident Reporting System (AIRS), and the Closed Claims Project (CCP).[41]

AQI developed NACOR and piloted the registry in 2010 with an initial cohort of six practices representing both academic university and private practice groups.[41] Participation in NACOR is for the primary purpose of supporting local practice quality improvement, through direct feedback of data to the individual practice and aggregation of data into external benchmarks that can be used to highlight areas for further review and allow comparison to other groups and facilities.[41, 43] NACOR participation is open to all anesthesia groups in the United States.

NACOR's data collection methodology differs from many registries that rely on case sampling and manual abstraction by reviewers by focusing on automated extraction of existing digital information.[41, 43, 44] Data is collected by periodic electronic reporting that is sent directly from each anesthesia practice to the registry.[41, 43, 45] The advantages of not relying on manual abstraction of data from medical records include both cost and time savings which reduce barriers to participation.[41, 43] The automated extraction of existing data and lack of reliance on manual data abstraction allows NACOR to aggregate data on a much larger number of cases; as of 2014, approximately 12 million total cases versus approximately 1.5 million total cases for NSQIP, which is based on sampling and data abstraction of major surgical cases at participating institutions.[41]

NACOR collects three "tiers" of data: a minimum dataset of demographic information extracted from billing software, immediate anesthesia clinical outcomes from the operating room and the postanesthesia care unit, and full reports from anesthesia information management systems, including intraoperative vital signs and medication doses.[42, 45] Accuracy and validity of data relies on a continuous process of multiple layers of both electronic and manual inspection.[43] Data is displayed via a detailed practice dashboard, and each participating anesthesia group has access to reports that illustrate trends over time and provide relevant national and peer group benchmarks.[43]

NACOR has created a sustainable and inclusive data registry that now has more than 30 million cases and is capturing data from approximately 33% of all anesthesia practices.[45] This large repository of anesthesia data has already supported multiple scientific publications.[45, 46, 47, 48, 49] One disadvantage of NACOR is that the registry remains voluntary, so there may be self-selection bias. Depending on the maturity of each anesthesia practice's automated information management system (AIMS), the practice may only be contributing data from their billing system and not the more detailed clinical outcomes and AIMS data.[45] Also, since AQI did not choose the data elements in NACOR but collected data that was available electronically, the data may be more heterogeneous in definition than those of other clinical registries.[43]

AQI also supports AIRS. AIRS solicits "any unintended event related to anesthesia or pain management with the significant potential for patient harm and captures both actual adverse events and near misses."[41] AIRS is the national equivalent of many of the voluntary incident reporting systems built by individual anesthesia departments. It allows for anonymous or confidential reporting of a specific event by any provider. It is intended to serve as an early warning system for clinical safety issues and to further AQI's educational activities.[41] Trends of common events are referred to AQI stakeholders – including sub-specialty societies, government agencies, and the Anesthesia Patient Safety Foundation – for action.[41] Since AIRS is a voluntary incident reporting system, it has similar advantages and disadvantages as anesthesia departmental incident reporting systems.

The Society for Pediatric Anesthesia developed Wake Up Safe (WUS), a national registry for reporting serious adverse events (SAEs) in pediatric anesthesia, for the purpose of quality improvement, using analysis of reported adverse events for learning.[21] Criteria for reporting an event include SAEs that occur during anesthesia or within 24 hours of the end of anesthesia care and are life threatening, result in death, or lead to prolonged hospitalization or disability. In addition, "never events," SAEs that should never happen to a patient (such as wrong site surgery or patient awareness), are captured by WUS. As of 2022, 38 major institutions participate in WUS, accounting for approximately 500,000 anesthetics per year.[50] WUS provides participating institutions with institution-specific demographic profiles and SAE reports that can be compared to participating institution averages for the purpose of benchmarking.[50]

Another important source of adverse event data is the Anesthesia Closed Claims Project (CCP) and its registry. The CCP works to identify safety concerns in anesthesia and patterns of injury, developing strategies for prevention of those events.[51] Data for this registry is gathered from closed malpractice cases involving anesthesiology providers. The CCP captures data from about half the malpractice insurance carriers in the United States.[41] Analysis of these events has shown important and previously unappreciated aspects of adverse anesthesia outcomes[52] and has led to numerous publications on the type of patients, situations, and events in anesthesia care that can result in adverse events and potential liability.[41]

Overall, national registries provide timely, actionable, and specific feedback to participating healthcare providers, enabling providers to understand their performance relative to their local and national peers.[36] The large number of cases in these registries is especially important in order to assess the risks of specific diseases, procedures, or patient populations, and allow calculation of incidence rates. One of the disadvantages of registries such as NACOR is that many anesthesia practices do not have EMRs or anesthesia information management systems that allow full participation. Another disadvantage is that there is currently no standard that defines how common data elements should be defined and captured in registries.[36]

Administrative Data

Existing electronic data such as admission and discharge data, billing data, and diagnostic codes from claims data can be searched for adverse events. The benefit of using this type of data is that one is able to review data from a large number of patients and compare that data across different healthcare settings.[1] However, since this data is usually collected for other purposes, the data is limited by accuracy of diagnostic coding and has been found to have relatively poor sensitivity and specificity for adverse event identification.[53] In 2015, Psaty et al. compared event rates and risk factor associations between reviewed hospitalized cardiovascular events and claims-based methods of defining events and found that conventional claims-based methods of defining events had high positive predictive values but low sensitivities.[54]

The Agency for Healthcare Research and Quality (AHRQ) developed a list of patient safety indicators using readily available hospital administrative data such as diagnosis and procedure codes.[1, 55, 56] These quality indicators are standardized, evidence-based measures of healthcare quality that can be used to measure and track clinical performance and outcomes over time and highlight potential areas for quality improvement.[55] PSIs place more emphasis on problems occurring in surgical and procedural practices, and detect fewer problems in medical or psychiatric patients.[5, 56] Multiple researchers have concluded that due to the variation in positive predictive value rates for many of the PSIs, they are best used as screening tools.[57]

Data from electronic medical resources like administrative data has multiple advantages, such as being cost-effective, readily available, and providing a substantial set of data on large patient populations. However, the drawbacks of this data source, such as lack of detailed clinical data and concerns over variability and inaccuracy of hospital coding across and within systems, make this a limited tool for identifying adverse events.[54, 56]

Automated Surveillance

The widespread use of EMR systems has allowed the development of automated surveillance systems to identify specifically defined events such as ADEs[31, 58] and hospital-acquired infections (HAIs).[59] Automated surveillance tools allow for the analysis of the vast amount of data in the EMR to identify adverse events within an individual healthcare system or across different healthcare systems.

Automated surveillance for ADEs was first demonstrated by Classen et al. in the early 1990s.[31, 58, 60] A computer program developed for the purpose of identifying ADEs was used to recognize combinations of clinical data that suggested a patient had suffered an ADE and to issue an alert.[31, 58] The computerized capture of an ADE reliably and reproducibly detected ADEs at a rate of four to ten times greater than voluntary reporting.[31, 58, 60] Since then, automated surveillance has been used for multiple other clinical applications.

The choice of data sources is an important consideration for creating automated surveillance programs. Valid and complete clinical data must be available and accessible via the information technology (IT) infrastructure. Administrative coding data (ACD) such as International Classification of Diseases (ICD) codes are attractive data points to use since they are easy to use and universally accepted across EMRs.[59] Though clinical data is considered more sensitive over time than administrative data alone, it may be difficult to extract the clinical information if the information resides in unstructured data fields. In addition, most EMRs use different information systems for laboratory, pharmacy, and billing systems, requiring an IT infrastructure that can create a format to retrieve and process the clinical data from different sources. The algorithms that use a combination of ACD and clinical data seem to be more reliable.[59]

The usefulness of automated surveillance has been limited, since many hospitals lack the IT infrastructure to support this methodology or lack the resources to evaluate the alerts generated.[60]

The algorithm of the automated surveillance system may range from a simple rule-based decision tree to multivariate regression models to machine learning. The specific algorithm employed depends on the purpose of the inquiry and the balancing of sensitivity and specificity. Computer algorithms combining diagnosis codes, microbiological analysis results, and antimicrobial medications have been used to identify HAIs with sensitivities and positive predictive values equivalent to conventional surveillance methods.[61]

Patient and Family Reported Adverse Events

Patient and family reported events are another source of data for identification of medical errors and associated adverse events. Involving the patient in reporting of events provides a direct benefit to the patient and captures adverse events that often have not been identified by any other hospital adverse event detection methods.[62, 63, 64] There is growing evidence that supports the feasibility and value of patient reported errors and adverse events.[65] Weissman found that patients reported twice as many adverse events than were identified during medical record review.[66] Multiple other studies have corroborated the finding that events reported by either patients or their families are often not captured by other reporting methodologies.[63, 67, 68, 69]

At present, patient and family reported adverse events are an infrequently utilized source of potential improvement data.[68] Standard practice should be to invite patients to report adverse events.[63] Gathering this information can be accomplished in several ways, including structured patient interviews during hospitalization, telephone surveys after discharge, and patient satisfaction surveys. Hospitals should incorporate questions about adverse events into patient satisfaction surveys.[65]

Since patient reporting is a relatively new method of collecting adverse event data, the most efficient technique with the highest yield of accurate data has not yet been defined.[62] Interviewing patients in person is an effective method to obtain high response rates (86–96%) from hospital patients.[63, 70]

Studies have shown that patients report adverse events accurately.[62, 63] Recall bias has been identified as a potential limitation.[62, 63] It can be minimized by ensuring that adverse events are documented as soon after the event as possible.[62] Using open-ended questions or asking for personal experiences will likely yield higher incident reporting rates[62, 63, 70] but requires more time to analyze the responses. Direct questions and limited response options allow for easier analysis but do not allow patients to share the details of the event.[62, 63, 70]

This approach could provide a sensitive and cost-effective quality improvement tool that yields data complementary to that generated by trigger tool-directed chart reviews and other adverse event collection methodology.[65] Patients also report nonsafety-related issues such as issues with communication, experience, staff interactions, care delivery, and hospital environment.[68] This type of data can be used to understand the overall patient experience and inform improvements. Patients are interested in engaging more in safety efforts and should be encouraged to take an active role in their healthcare. If patients are asked to take a more active role in their care and are able to identify errors, they may be able to intercept errors before harm occurs.[63]

Summary

A number of specific methods to identify and measure medical errors and adverse events have been described. Provider-initiated incident reports can be easily collected and engage frontline personnel to identify both adverse events and near misses. However, this method is limited by the voluntary nature of provider reporting that can lead to significant under-reporting or a selection bias in which events are reported. Retrospective chart reviews, though long considered the gold standard for identifying adverse events, are labor- and time-intensive, making retrospective chart reviews less practical for large-scale implementation. Trigger tool methodology allows for more consistent and accurate identification and tracking of adverse events since it is independent of voluntary reporting by providers.

The challenge in using trigger tool methodology is defining the specific trigger to identify the adverse event. Clinical national registries that collect data from across healthcare systems allow for assessment of risks for specific diseases, procedures, or patient populations, as well as enabling providers to understand their performance relative to their local and national peers by providing benchmarking data. The difficulty with clinical registries is in determining standards for how data elements are defined and captured. Existing data from administrative data such as diagnostic codes and billing data can be a cost-effective and easily accessible source of information for adverse events. However, this method is limited by lack of detailed clinical data and inaccuracies in coding data. Automated surveillance in EMRs can be used to identify specifically defined adverse events by analyzing multiple data sources within the EMR. Though this method offers much promise, it requires a sophisticated IT infrastructure to build and maintain the algorithms. Finally, patients and families are accurate sources for reporting events and may be a sensitive and cost-effective method for identifying both adverse events and near misses.

Despite the multiple methods described above to identify adverse events, there is no ideal, nationally agreed-upon measurement strategy.[1, 53] A study by Naessens to determine whether an adverse event could be identified by different methods found that each method identified different adverse events and very few adverse events were identified by multiple methods.[5] These results suggest using more than one method of identifying patient harm so as to better capture any possible patient safety issues.[1, 5, 71]

There is also the need to move from nonsystematic methods such as voluntary reporting to coordinated systematic measurements.[1] A coordinated systematic approach to data collection of adverse events via EMRs would allow for data comparison across healthcare systems to inform national incidence rates of adverse events. Defining national incidence rates of events is particularly important for rare events that occur in the context of small patient populations. Implementation and growth of the electronic health record may provide an opportunity to launch a national standardized reporting structure.[53]

References

1. Rafter N, Hickey A, Condell S, et al. Adverse events in healthcare: Learning from mistakes. *QJM*. 2015;108(4):273–277. doi: 10.1093/qjmed/hcu145 [published Online First: 2014/08/01].

2. Resar RK, Rozich JD, and Classen D. Methodology and rationale for the measurement of harm with trigger tools. *Quality & Safety in Health Care*. 2003;12(Suppl 2):ii39–45. [published Online First: 2003/12/04].

3. Stockwell DC, Bisarya H, Classen DC, et al. A trigger tool to detect harm in pediatric inpatient settings. *Pediatrics*. 2015;135(6):1036–1042. doi: 10.1542/peds.2014-2152 [published Online First: 2015/05/20].

4. Levtzion-Korach O, Frankel A, Alcalai H, et al. Integrating incident data from five reporting systems to assess patient safety: making sense of the elephant. *Joint Commission Journal on Quality and Patient Safety*. 2010;36(9):402–410. [published Online First: 2010/09/30].

5. Naessens JM, Campbell CR, Huddleston JM, et al. A comparison of hospital adverse events identified by three widely used detection methods. *International Journal of Quality Health Care*. 2009;21(4):301–307. doi: 10.1093/intqhc/mzp027 [published Online First: 2009/07/21].

6. Kohn LT, Corrigan JM, and Donaldson MS, eds. *To Err is Human. Institute of Medicine (US) Committee on Quality of Health Care in America*. Washington, DC, National Academies Press, 2000. Available from www.ncbi.nlm.nih.gov/books/NBK225174/ (Accessed 7/10/22).

7. Leonard MS. Patient safety and quality improvement: medical errors and adverse events. *Pediatrics in Review* 2010;31(4):151–158. doi: 10.1542/pir.31-4-151 [published Online First: 2010/04/03].

8. Griffin FA RR. *IHI global Trigger Tool for Measuring Adverse Events (Second Edition).* IHI Innovation Series White Paper. Cambridge, MA, Institute for Healthcare Improvement; 2009.

9. Jick H. Drugs--remarkably nontoxic. *New England Journal of Medicine.* 1974;291(16):824–828. doi: 10.1056/NEJM197410172911605 [published Online First: 1974/10/17].

10. Leape LL. Errors in medicine. *Clinica Chimica Acta.* 2009;404(1):2–5. doi: 10.1016/j.cca.2009.03.020 [published Online First: 2009/03/24].

11. Leape LL, Brennan TA, Laird N, et al. The nature of adverse events in hospitalized patients. Results of the Harvard Medical Practice Study II. *New England Journal of Medicine.* 1991;324(6):377–384. doi: 10.1056/NEJM199102073240605 [published Online First: 1991/02/07].

12. Staender S. Incident reporting in anaesthesiology. *Best Practice and Research in Clinical Anaesthesiology.* 2011;25(2):207–214. doi: 10.1016/j.bpa.2011.01.005 [published Online First: 2011/05/10].

13. Guffey PJ, Culwick M, and Merry AF. Incident reporting at the local and national level. *International Anesthesiology Clinics.* 2014;52(1):69–83. Doi: 10.1097/AIA.0000000000000008 [published Online First: 2013/12/29].

14. Flanagan JC. The critical incident technique. *Psychological Bulletin.* 1954;51(4):327–358. [published Online First: 1954/07/01].

15. Cooper JB, Newbower RS, Long CD, et al. Preventable anesthesia mishaps: A study of human factors. *Anesthesiology.* 1978;49(6):399–406. [published Online First: 1978/12/01].

16. Williams GD, Muffly MK, Mendoza JM, et al. Reporting of perioperative adverse events by pediatric anesthesiologists at a Tertiary Children's Hospital: Targeted interventions to increase the rate of reporting. *Anesthesia and Analgesia.* 2017;125(5):1515–1523. doi: 10.1213/ANE.0000000000002208 [published Online First: 2017/07/06].

17. Farley DO, Haviland A, Champagne S, et al. Adverse-event-reporting practices by US hospitals: Results of a national survey. *Quality & Safety in Health Care.* 2008;17(6):416–423. doi: 10.1136/qshc.2007.024638 [published Online First: 2008/12/10].

18. Haller G, Courvoisier DS, Anderson H, et al. Clinical factors associated with the non-utilization of an anaesthesia incident reporting system. *British Journal of Anaesthesia.* 2011;107(2):171–179. doi: 10.1093/bja/aer148 [published Online First: 2011/06/07].

19. Peterfreund RA, Driscoll WD, Walsh JL, et al. Evaluation of a mandatory quality assurance data capture in anesthesia: A secure electronic system to capture quality assurance information linked to an automated anesthesia record. *Anesthesia and Analgesia.* 2011;112(5):1218–1225. doi: 10.1213/ANE.0b013e31821207f0 [published Online First: 2011/03/19].

20. Larizgoitia I, Bouesseau MC, and Kelley E. WHO efforts to promote reporting of adverse events and global learning. *Journal of Public Health Research.* 2013;2(3):e29. doi: 10.4081/jphr.2013.e29 [published Online First: 2014/08/30].

21. Tjia I, Rampersad S, Varughese A, et al. Wake Up Safe and root cause analysis: Quality improvement in pediatric anesthesia. *Anesthesia and Analgesia.* 2014;119(1):122–136. doi: 10.1213/ANE.0000000000000266 [published Online First: 2014/06/20].

22. Rowin EJ, Lucier D, Pauker SG, et al. Does error and adverse event reporting by physicians and nurses differ? *Joint Commission Journal of Quality and Patient Safety.* 2008;34(9):537–545. [published Online First: 2008/09/17].

23. Heard GC, Sanderson PM, and Thomas RD. Barriers to adverse event and error reporting in anesthesia. *Anesthesia and Analgesia.* 2012;114(3):604–614. doi: 10.1213/ANE.0b013e31822649e8 [published Online First: 2011/08/09].

24. Mahajan RP. Critical incident reporting and learning. *British Journal of Anaesthesia.* 2010;105(1):69–75. doi: 10.1093/bja/aeq133 [published Online First: 2010/06/17].

25. Guffey P, Szolnoki J, Caldwell J, et al. Design and implementation of a near-miss reporting system at a large, academic pediatric anesthesia department. *Paediatric Anaesthesia.* 2011;21(7):810–814. doi: 10.1111/j.1460-9592.2011.03574.x [published Online First: 2011/05/04].

26. Murff HJ, Patel VL, Hripcsak G, et al. Detecting adverse events for patient safety research: A review of current methodologies. *Journal of Biomedical Informatics.* 2003;36(1–2):131–143. [published Online First: 2003/10/14].

27. Brennan TA, Leape LL, Laird NM, et al. Incidence of adverse events and negligence in hospitalized patients. Results of the Harvard Medical Practice Study I. *New England Journal of Medicine.* 1991;324(6):370–376. doi: 10.1056/NEJM199102073240604 [published Online First: 1991/02/07].

28. Hiatt HH, Barnes BA, Brennan TA, et al. A study of medical injury and medical malpractice. *New England Journal of Medicine.* 1989;321(7):480–484. doi: 10.1056/NEJM198908173210725 [published Online First: 1989/08/17].

29. Baker GR, Norton PG, Flintoft V, et al. The Canadian Adverse Events Study: The incidence of adverse events among hospital patients in Canada. *CMAJ.* 2004;170(11):1678–1686. [published Online First: 2004/05/26].

30. Classen DC, Lloyd RC, Provost L, et al. Development and evaluation of the Institute for Healthcare Improvement Global Trigger Tool. 2008;4(3):169–177. doi: 10.1097/PTS.0b013e318183a475.

31. Classen DC, Pestotnik SL, Evans RS, et al. Description of a computerized adverse drug event monitor using a hospital information system. *Hospital Pharmacy.* 1992;27(9):774, 76–79, 83. [published Online First: 1992/09/01].

32. Classen DC, Resar R, Griffin F, et al. "Global trigger tool" shows that adverse events in hospitals may be ten times greater than previously measured. *Health Affairs (Millwood).* 2011;30(4):581–589. doi: 10.1377/hlthaff.2011.0190 [published Online First: 2011/04/08].

33. Howe CL. A review of the Office of Inspector General's reports on adverse event identification and reporting. *Journal of Healthcare Risk Management.* 2011;30(4):48–54. doi: 10.1002/jhrm.20068 [published Online First: 2011/04/21].

34. Rutberg H, Borgstedt Risberg M, Sjodahl R, et al. Characterisations of adverse events detected in a university hospital: A 4-year study using the Global Trigger Tool method. *BMJ Open.* 2014;4(5):e004879. doi: 10.1136/bmjopen-2014-004879 [published Online First: 2014/05/30].

35. Sharek PJ and Classen D. The incidence of adverse events and medical error in pediatrics. *Pediatric Clinics of North America.* 2006;53(6):1067–1077. doi: 10.1016/j.pcl.2006.09.011 [published Online First: 2006/11/28].

36. Blumenthal S. The use of clinical registries in the United States: A landscape survey. *EGEMS (Washington DC).* 2017;5(1):26. doi: 10.5334/egems.248 [published Online First: 2018/06/23].

37. Hall BL, Hamilton BH, Richards K, et al. Does surgical quality improve in the American College of Surgeons National Surgical Quality Improvement Program: An evaluation of all participating hospitals. *Annals of Surgery.* 2009;250(3):363–376. doi: 10.1097/SLA.0b013e3181b4148f [published Online First: 2009/08/01].

38. Khuri SF. The NSQIP: A new frontier in surgery. *Surgery.* 2005;138(5):837–843. doi: 10.1016/j.surg.2005.08.016 [published Online First: 2005/11/18].

39. Khuri SF, Daley J, Henderson W, et al. The Department of Veterans Affairs' NSQIP: The first national, validated, outcome-based, risk-adjusted, and peer-controlled program for the measurement and enhancement of the quality of surgical care. National VA Surgical Quality Improvement Program. *Annals of*

Surgery. 1998;228(4):491–507. [published Online First: 1998/10/28]

40. Khuri SF, Henderson WG, Daley J, et al. Successful implementation of the Department of Veterans Affairs' National Surgical Quality Improvement Program in the private sector: The Patient Safety in Surgery study. *Annals of Surgery*. 2008;248(2):329–336. doi: 10.1097/SLA.0b013e3181823485 [published Online First: 2008/07/25].

41. Dutton RP. Registries of the anesthesia quality institute. *International Anesthesiology Clinics*. 2014;52(1):1–14. doi: 10.1097/AIA.0000000000000001 [published Online First: 2013/12/29].

42. Dutton RP and Dukatz A. Quality improvement using automated data sources: The anesthesia quality institute. *Anesthesiology Clinics*. 2011;29(3):439–454. doi: 10.1016/j.anclin.2011.05.002 [published Online First: 2011/08/30].

43. Liau A, Havidich JE, Onega T, et al. The National Anesthesia Clinical Outcomes Registry. *Anesthesia and Analgesia*. 2015;121(6):1604–1610. doi: 10.1213/ane.0000000000000895 [published Online First: 2015/11/19].

44. Thomas EG, Andrew D, Hubert AK, et al. Bring Out Your Data: The Evolution of the National Anesthesia Clinical Outcomes Registry (NACOR). *International Journal of Computational Models and Algorithms in Medicine (IJCMAM)*. 2011;2(2):51–69. doi: 10.4018/jcmam.2011040104.

45. Dutton RP. Large databases in anaesthesiology. *Current Opinion in Anaesthesiology*. 2015;28(6):697–702. doi: 10.1097/ACO.0000000000000243 [published Online First: 2015/09/30].

46. Deiner S, Westlake B, and Dutton RP. Patterns of surgical care and complications in elderly adults. *Journal of the American Geriatrics Society*. 2014;62(5):829–835. doi: 10.1111/jgs.12794 [published Online First: 2014/04/16].

47. Dexter F, Dutton RP, Kordylewski H, et al. Anesthesia workload nationally during regular workdays and weekends. *Anesthesia and Analgesia*.

2015;121(6):1600–1603. doi: 10.1213/ANE.0000000000000773 [published Online First: 2015/04/30].

48. Nunnally ME, O'Connor MF, Kordylewski H, et al. The incidence and risk factors for perioperative cardiac arrest observed in the national anesthesia clinical outcomes registry. *Anesthesia and Analgesia*. 2015;120(2):364–370. doi: 10.1213/ANE.0000000000000527 [published Online First: 2014/11/13].

49. Shapiro FE, Jani SR, Liu X, et al. Initial results from the National Anesthesia Clinical Outcomes Registry and overview of office-based anesthesia. *Anesthesiology Clinics*. 2014;32(2):431–444. doi: 10.1016/j.anclin.2014.02.018 [published Online First: 2014/06/03].

50. Wake Up Safe. Available from: http://wakeupsafe.org/ (Accessed 27/01/2019).

51. Anesthesia Closed Claims Project. [cited 2019 January 27]. Available from: https://depts.washington.edu/asaccp/welcome-anesthesia-closed-claims-project-its-registries.

52. Cheney FW. The American Society of Anesthesiologists Closed Claims Project: What have we learned, how has it affected practice, and how will it affect practice in the future? *Anesthesiology*. 1999;91(2):552–556. [published Online First: 1999/08/12].

53. Jha AK and Classen DC. Getting moving on patient safety–harnessing electronic data for safer care. *New England Journal of Medicine*. 2011;365(19):1756–1758. doi: 10.1056/NEJMp1109398 [published Online First: 2011/11/11].

54. Psaty BM, Delaney JA, Arnold AM, et al. Study of cardiovascular health outcomes in the era of claims data: The Cardiovascular Health Study. *Circulation*. 2016;133(2):156–164. doi: 10.1161/CIRCULATIONAHA.115.018610 [published Online First: 2015/11/06].

55. Agency for Healthcare Research and Quality. AHRQ Quality Indicators]. Available from: www.qualityindicators.ahrq.gov (Accessed 7/10/2022).

56. Farquhar M. Chapter 45: AHRQ Quality Indicators. In: Hughes RG, ed. *Patient*

Safety and Quality: An Evidence-Based Handbook for Nurses. Rockville, MD, Agency for Healthcare Research and Quality (US), April 2008.

57. Narain W. Assessing estimates of patient safety derived from coded data. Journal of Healthcare Quality. 2017;39(4):230–242. doi: 10.1097/JHQ.0000000000000088 [published Online First: 2017/06/29].

58. Classen DC, Pestotnik SL, Evans RS, et al. Computerized surveillance of adverse drug events in hospital patients. JAMA. 1991;266(20):2847–2851. [published Online First: 1991/11/27].

59. Sips ME, Bonten MJM, and van Mourik MSM. Automated surveillance of healthcare-associated infections: State of the art. Current Opinion in Infectious Diseases. 2017;30(4):425–431. Doi: 10.1097/QCO.0000000000000376 [published Online First: 2017/05/16].

60. Kilbridge PM and Classen DC. Automated surveillance for adverse events in hospitalized patients: Back to the future. Quality & Safety in Health Care. 2006;15(3):148–149. doi: 10.1136/qshc.2006.018218 [published Online First: 2006/06/06].

61. Klompas M and Yokoe DS. Automated surveillance of health care-associated infections. Clinical Infectious Disease. 2009;48(9):1268–1275. doi: 10.1086/597591 [published Online First: 2009/04/02].

62. King A, Daniels J, Lim J, et al. Time to listen: a review of methods to solicit patient reports of adverse events. Quality & Safety in Health Care. 2010;19(2):148–157. doi: 10.1136/qshc.2008.030114 [published Online First: 2010/03/31].

63. Weingart SN, Pagovich O, Sands DZ, et al. What can hospitalized patients tell us about adverse events? Learning from patient-reported incidents. Journal of General Internal Medicine. 2005;20(9):830–836. doi: 10.1111/j.1525-1497.2005.0180.x [published Online First: 2005/08/25].

64. Zhu J, Stuver SO, Epstein AM, et al. Can we rely on patients' reports of adverse events? Medical Care. 2011;49(10):948–955. doi: 10.1097/MLR.0b013e31822047a8 [published Online First: 2011/06/07].

65. Weingart SN. Patient-reported adverse events: What are we waiting for? Joint Commission Journal on Quality & Patient Safety. 2011;37(11):494. [published Online First: 2011/12/03].

66. Weissman JS, Schneider EC, Weingart SN, et al. Comparing patient-reported hospital adverse events with medical record review: Do patients know something that hospitals do not? Annals of Internal Medicine. 2008;149(2):100–108. [published Online First: 2008/07/16].

67. Hasegawa T, Fujita S, Seto K, et al. Patients' identification and reporting of unsafe events at six hospitals in Japan. Joint Commission Journal on Quality & Patient Safety. 2011;37(11):502–508. [published Online First: 2011/12/03].

68. Khan A, Furtak SL, Melvin P, et al. Parent-reported errors and adverse events in hospitalized children. JAMA Pediatrics. 2016;170(4):e154608. doi: 10.1001/jamapediatrics.2015.4608 [published Online First: 2016/03/02].

69. Ohrn A, Elfstrom J, Liedgren C, et al. Reporting of sentinel events in Swedish hospitals: A comparison of severe adverse events reported by patients and providers. Joint Commission Journal on Quality & Patient Safety. 2011;37(11):495–501. [published Online First: 2011/12/03].

70. Weingart SN, Price J, Duncombe D, et al. Patient-reported safety and quality of care in outpatient oncology. Joint Commission Journal on Quality & Patient Safety. 2007;33(2):83–94. [published Online First: 2007/03/21].

71. Olsen S, Neale G, Schwab K, et al. Hospital staff should use more than one method to detect adverse events and potential adverse events: Incident reporting, pharmacist surveillance and local real-time record review may all have a place. Quality & Safety in Health Care. 2007;16(1):40–44. doi: 10.1136/qshc.2005.017616 [published Online First: 2007/02/16].

Chapter 8

Learning from Adverse Events: Classification Systems

Imelda M. Tjia and Nathaniel Greene

Classification Systems

Introduction

"Medicine used to be simple ... effective and dangerous."[1] With the evolution of medical technology and increased specialization, there are many moments in which incidents can occur that can compromise patient safety. Patient safety reporting systems should be designed to facilitate healthcare systems to learn from these failures in order to improve patient safety.[2] Healthcare organizations strive to deliver the safest and best patient care, and organizations should learn best practices from each other. However, different healthcare organizations have different reporting systems with different terminologies, data fields, and classifications; therefore, establishing a uniform reporting system across all healthcare organizations is a tremendous challenge.[3] The use of a standardized classification system for adverse events would help healthcare organizations disseminate information and develop a common language for medical events.[4]

Creation of a standardized classification system

A classification system, or a taxonomy, provides an "organizing framework" and "degree of analytical insight into the way errors and adverse events are discussed and 'managed' within the context of health care governance."[5] On a more abstract level, the structure of a taxonomy evolved from principles founded by the empiricists and the organizational rationalists.[5]

The empiricists track information regarding the type, location, and frequency of the error. This basic data will reveal if an organization is effectively reducing errors.[5] Organizational rationalists examine and evaluate the organizations as systems in which the errors occur using "cognitive psychology, human factors research and the sociology of organizations."[5] Cognitive psychologists Rasmussen and Jensen use a skill-rule-knowledge theory to explain errors. This theory elucidates that a person committing a "skill-based error" has the appropriate skills and experience, but a memory lapse may have led to the error. A "rule-based error" is the result of incorrect action due to disregard of certain rules or policies. "Knowledge-based errors" are the consequence of an individual's insufficient knowledge leading to adverse events.[5]

In a complex organization, the structure may be composed of many different layers. Reason describes the difference between latent and active failures in a complex system. Active failures are errors that occur in direct contact with the patient, involving slips, mistakes, and rule-violating activity committed by those at the "sharp end" of organizational systems and have immediate adverse consequences.[5] Conversely, errors that are a result of failures in the system (i.e., poor staffing, malfunctioning equipment), or the "blunt end," are known as latent failures.[5]

The World Health Organization (WHO) constructed a specific taxonomy for medical errors around an adverse event, naming it "the Incident type" and categorizing its contributing factors, patient characteristics, and outcomes of that specific event; the taxonomy also classifies mitigating and preventative actions for that event.[6] Taking this approach allows healthcare institutions to learn many lessons from other fields such as aviation and other high-risk industries as they have been influential in advancing the reporting, analysis, and classification of adverse events.[7]

Medication error taxonomies

The aforementioned high-risk industries have pioneered the way in reducing errors "by applying human factors engineering, a discipline that designs ... systems, and policies to increase worker efficiency and decrease human errors."[8] Because human factors are such a big part of the complex system of healthcare, it is critical to reduce errors to decrease the number of adverse events resulting from human error. It is important to understand the environment in which the healthcare provider is working and the pressures that he encounters that impact his judgment and decision-making processes.[8] A medication error is an example of a situation in which human factors may play a fundamental role.

The National Coordinating Council for Medication Error Reporting and Prevention (NCC MERP) released a medication error taxonomy in 1999 that provided "a standard language and structure ... to be used to develop databases to analyze medication errors and organized them into eight major categories: (1) patient information, (2) medication error event, (3) patient outcome, (4) product information, (5) personnel information, (6) type of medication error, (7) causes, and (8) contributing factors."[8]

The NCC MERP taxonomy proved to be useful for collecting certain data as it does focus on human factors, such as insufficient training or user error. However, the classification system did not facilitate the categorization of errors. This reporting system relied mostly on free text, and the format made the analysis of events difficult.[8] Reporting systems should not only be databases of adverse events. Healthcare organizations should use the collected information to detect problems and create solutions to prevent recurrence of these events that compromise patient care.

Primary care taxonomies

A classification system of adverse events designed specifically for primary care practices may have unique components that may not be found in other classification systems.[9] Primary care practices will evaluate the healthcare system in which the patient is receiving care that may have led to the incident that compromised patient care: delay in treatment, process errors, clinician factors (judgment, skills), communication factors (clinicians, patients), administration factors (clinician, pharmacy, ancillary providers), and blunt end factors (insurance company regulations, governmental regulations, size and location of the practice). Additionally, it is important to list patient risk factors that led to adverse events. Was there a language barrier that prevented the patient from understanding the provider's instructions? Elder et al. explain that adding the patient's perspective to the taxonomy is significant because changes can be made to improve patient factors such as language translators and reminder phone calls. The consideration of all contributing factors, including patient factors, resulting in adverse events that compromise patient care in the taxonomy will make the analysis comprehensive and help prevent recurrence of those events in the future.

Key components of a classification system

When designing a classification system, users must propose a taxonomy that can be used for all events (actual and near miss) and all medical specialties (ambulatory care, surgery, medicine, etc.). While providers typically learn from actual events where they were aware of patient harm taking place, there is usually less impact from "near-miss" events unless properly reviewed with the appropriate actions taken in response. Additionally, terminology of any taxonomy should be commonly used. Usability of the taxonomies should be easy and universal for clinicians, researchers, malpractice insurers, and accreditation and regulatory bodies. Taxonomies should also enable organizations to categorize contributory factors (i.e., "underlying failures in knowledge and culture, physical structure, business processes, human behavior and factors, hazardous conditions") and include impact of the events, corrective actions, and likelihood for recurrence.

Two such taxonomies have come to the forefront and are in use today by healthcare institutions across the United States: the Healthcare Performance Improvement (HPI) Safety Event Classification (SEC) and the Joint Commission (JC) formerly known as the Joint Commission on the Accreditation of Healthcare Organizations (JCAHO) Patient Safety Taxonomy. Developed by independent organizations, these taxonomies approach patient safety events in different ways and are complementary to one another in several aspects.

HPI taxonomy

The HPI SEC derives its foundation from separating "harm" from "bad outcomes." Fundamentally, a safety event is an occurrence where there has been a deviation from generally accepted performance standards (GAPS), and there is a direct cause and effect relationship between this deviation and the occurrence. This occurrence is then further characterized into one of three categories depending on whether the event reached a patient, and if it did, the degree of harm to that patient from the particular event (Figure 8.1).

This taxonomy establishes that if there is an unfavorable outcome with no deviation from GAPS, no safety event has occurred. If a deviation from GAPS occurred that did not reach the patient, this is classified as a "near miss" safety event. Depending on how this safety event is identified, these near miss safety events are further classified into an early barrier catch (caught by initial safety barrier as planned), a last strong barrier catch (missed by previous safety barrier mechanisms and caught by final barrier in place), or an unplanned catch (no planned safety barrier, just caught by random chance). This further classification allows the impact of near miss events to be educational and inform the system on how to prevent such occurrences in the future without any patient harm. If patient harm has occurred, this taxonomy then classifies events as a serious safety event if the event caused moderate or severe harm (whether it is temporary or permanent) or death. If the event caused minimal, no detectable harm, or no harm, the event is then classified as a precursor safety event.

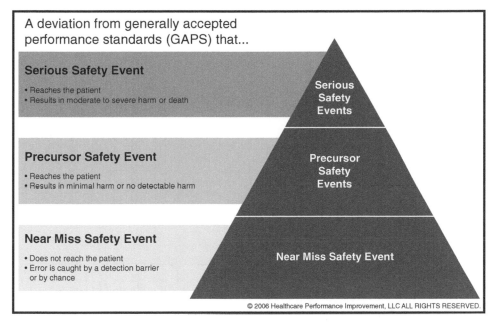

A deviation from generally accepted performance standards (GAPS) that...

Serious Safety Event
- Reaches the patient
- Results in moderate to severe harm or death

Serious Safety Events

Precursor Safety Event
- Reaches the patient
- Results in minimal harm or no detectable harm

Precursor Safety Events

Near Miss Safety Event
- Does not reach the patient
- Error is caught by a detection barrier or by chance

Near Miss Safety Event

Figure 8.1 HPI Structural Approach to Safety Events Classification. Reproduced with permission from Press Ganey "used with permission from Press Ganey Healthcare Performance Improvement (HPI). Copyright 2018" (A black and white version of this figure will appear in some formats. For the color version, refer to the plate section.)

The HPI SEC goes further to classify deviations from GAPS by investigating "failure modes" both at the level of the individual and the overall system. This further classification can help identify the factors (sometimes multiple) that led to a particular safety event and both help inform how to improve the system and the individual. Root causes of events nearly always are found as deficiencies in organizational systems.[10]

In addition to analysis of the causes and severity of events, the HPI taxonomy also has created a system to categorize events in an effort to combine topic areas of similar events to be informative to different areas of the healthcare environment (Figure 8.2).

Events can generally be categorized into one of six areas: procedural, environmental, patient protection, care management, product or device, or criminal. This type of categorization allows for healthcare institutions to identify and track particular care areas over time and understand how effective safety interventions developed as a result of particular events are.

This taxonomy provides a framework to create a meaningful metric over time that hospitals can measure (and report) to inform and benchmark their particular safety culture. This measure is called the "serious safety event rate" and is measured by counting the number of serious safety events in the past 12 months and dividing by the relevant number of "adjusted patient days" in the last 12 months. An institution could develop this metric with regard to the entire system or within a specific category to better understand the overall performance of their institution.

The HPI SEC employs a unique approach to addressing patient safety while giving users impactful tools to create and strengthen institutional safety culture. While the HPI SEC is a commonly used approach, many institutions use an additional (or sometimes different) approach to further strengthen their safety culture.

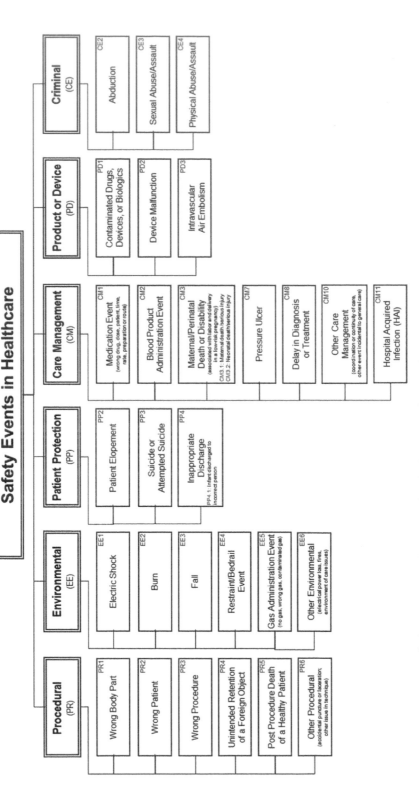

Figure 8.2 HPI Taxonomy of Safety Events in Healthcare. Reproduced with *permission from Press Ganey* "used with permission from Press Ganey Healthcare Performance Improvement (HPI). Copyright 2018." (A black and white version of this figure will appear in some formats. For the color version, refer to the plate section.)

The Joint Commission taxonomy

As the WHO taxonomy of adverse events categorizes the contributing factors, patient characteristics, and outcomes of the specific event as well as the mitigating and preventative actions for the event, the JC patient safety taxonomy utilizes the following five primary classifications[11]:

(1) **Impact**: the outcome or effects of medical error and systems failure, commonly referred to as "harm to the patient"
(2) **Type**: the implied or visible processes that were faulty or failed
(3) **Domain**: the characteristics of the setting in which the incident occurred and the type of individuals involved
(4) **Cause**: the factors and agents that led to the incident
(5) **Prevention and mitigation**: the measures taken or proposed to reduce incidence and effects of adverse occurrences

The JC taxonomy defines the patient's outcome resulting from the error by classifying *impact* (Figure 8.3) which is divided into two harm categories: medical (psychological or physical) and nonmedical (legal, social, or economic). Furthermore, the resulting harm is characterized from varying degrees ranging from no harm to mild harm to permanent harm.

Contributing factors leading to the event can be identified by the *type* classification (Figure 8.4) which detects process breakdowns that involve communication, patient management, or clinical performance. Communication problems may "exist between provider and patient, provider and patient's proxy, provider and non-medical staff and among providers," such as hierarchical problems in surgical teams.[11] Examples of patient management failures include "improper delegation, failure in tracking or follow-up, wrong referral or consultation, or questionable use of resources."[11] Problems with clinical performance may include "iatrogenic events during the pre-intervention, intervention and post-intervention phases of care" such as suboptimal training procedures or failure to mark operative sites preoperatively.[11]

Patient characteristics of an adverse event are described by the *domain* classification (Figure 8.5) of the JC taxonomy. The patient's age, gender, diagnosis, coexisting conditions, race, ethnicity, education level, and disease duration are classified under *domain*. This classification also identifies the healthcare setting (i.e., hospital, physician office, ambulatory care setting, nursing home) in which the event evolved, frequently including the general hospital (64%), psychiatric hospital (13%), psychiatric unit (6%), outpatient behavioral health (5%), emergency department (4%), long-term facility care (4%), home care service (3%), and ambulatory care setting (1.5%).[11] Additionally, the *domain* classification defines the staff involved in the event: physician, dentist, health profession student, nurse, therapist, pharmacist or other caregiver. Intended patient care intervention (i.e., therapeutic, diagnostic, rehabilitative, preventative, palliative, research) is also delineated under the *domain* classification.

The *cause* (Figure 8.6) of adverse events can be attributed to system failures or to human failures. Problems in "design, organization, training or maintenance that lead to operator errors"[11] are considered system failures. System failures are analogous to latent failures. Conversely, human failures are skill or knowledge deficiencies, failure to comply with policy and procedures, or other factors on the part of the clinician. Human failures are comparable to active failures.

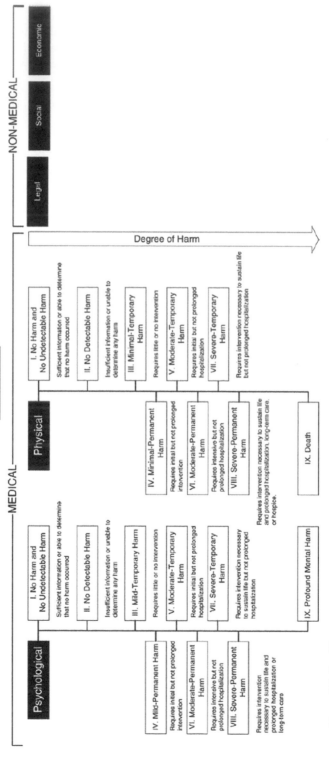

Figure 8.3 The JC impact taxonomy

All Joint Commission taxonomies, reproduced with permission from Rights Link November 17, 2020.

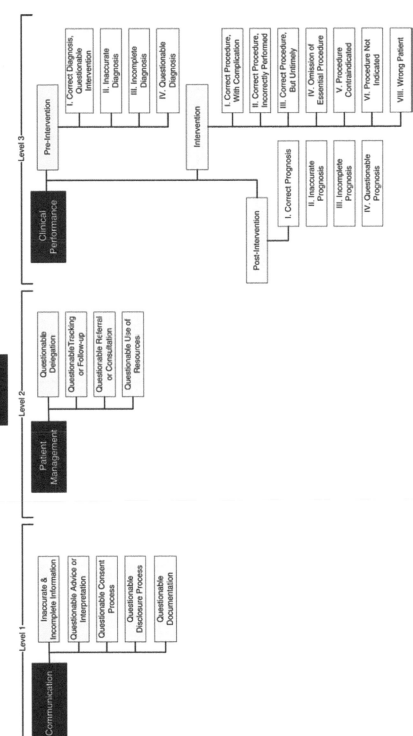

Figure 8.4 The JC type taxonomy

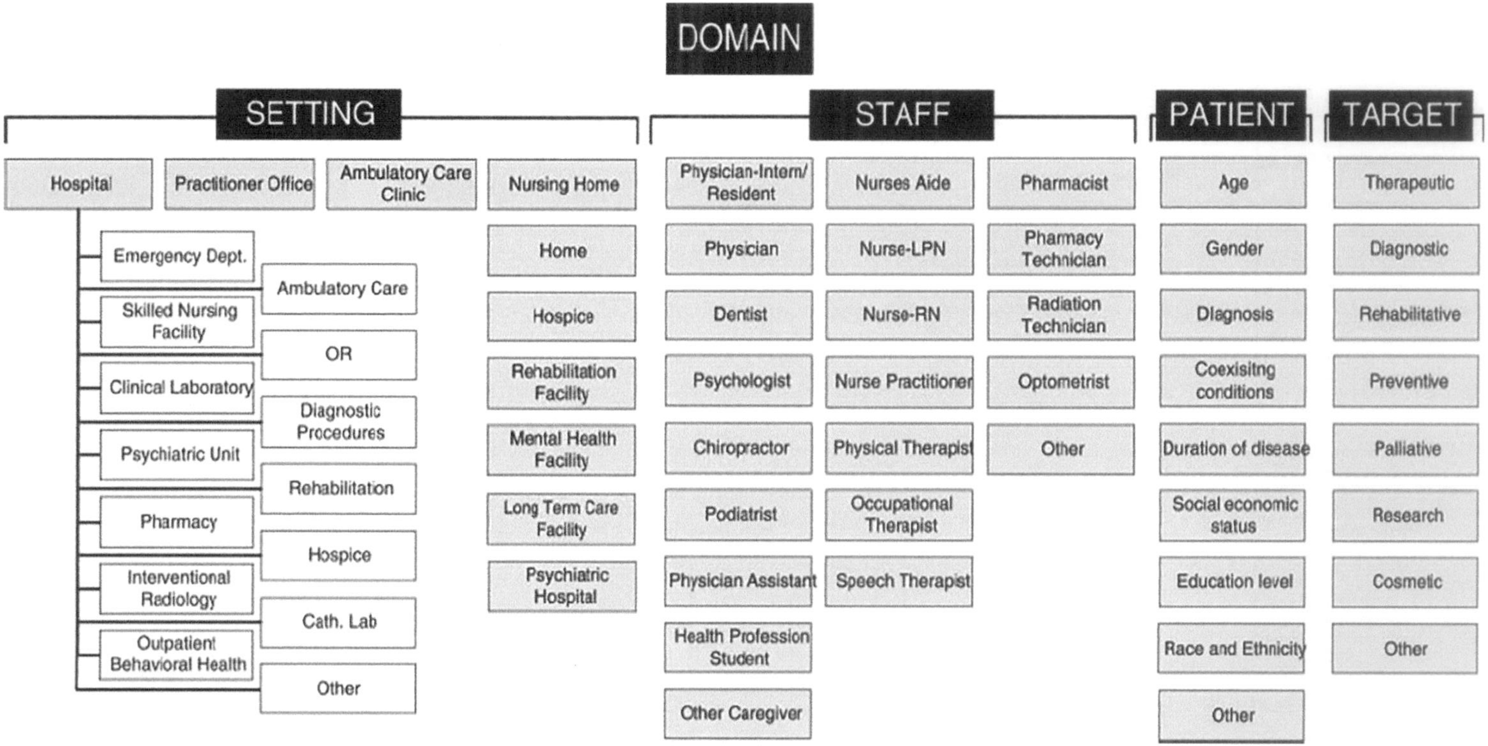

Figure 8.5 The JC domain taxonomy

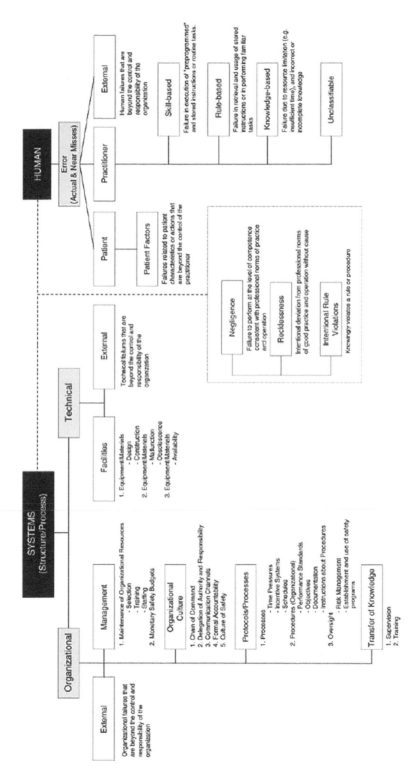

Figure 8.6 The JC cause taxonomy

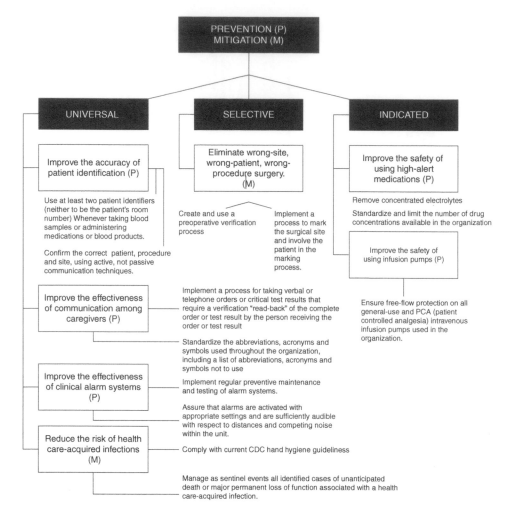

Figure 8.7 The JC prevention and mitigation taxonomy

The final taxonomy, ***prevention and mitigation*** (Figure 8.7), identifies causes that have resulted in system failures and adverse events and proposes processes and strategies that will prevent those failures from reoccurring. Examples of specific actions in this classification used to mitigate adverse events include accurate patient identification, effective communication between caregivers, effective use of clinical alarm systems, and preoperative surgical site marking to prevent wrong-site surgery.

The patient safety event taxonomy could "be used as a common backbone when mapped to disparate reporting systems unifying terminologies and classifications … [allowing] aggregated data to be combined and tracked over time, [providing] consistency across reporting systems, and [structuring] data documentation and presentation using a standardized format. Applied to an electronic health record system, the taxonomy offers a means for interoperability, facilitating exchange of patient safety data across systems."[11] The challenges of using this taxonomy include the possibility that events may not be classifiable using this system. An event may be too complicated to classify or code in a simple taxonomy.

The Joint Commission and HPI taxonomy similarities and differences

While current event taxonomies are "categorical classifications in that events are identified by event type, such as wrong site procedure, fall with injury, or burn, the HPI SEC is an outcome-based classification system.... The event is assessed for defects in care, or deviations from GAPS; a direct cause-and-effect relationship between deviations and the outcome, and … the safety event is classified according to level of patient harm resulting from the event."[12]

Just as the JC taxonomy classifies patient harm, the HPI method has a similar classification system: both were based upon the NCC MERP taxonomy. The JC taxonomy differentiates impact by medical and nonmedical harm; the HPI method distinguishes the same levels of harm (no harm, no detectable harm, minimal to severe harm, and temporary to permanent harm) by the specific safety event (near miss, precursor, or serious safety event).[12]

As the JC taxonomy identifies the process breakdown (communication, patient management, and clinical performance) by classifying the *type* of event, HPI's Taxonomy of Safety Events in Healthcare identifies the nature of the events through the following categories: procedural, environmental, patient protection, care management, product device, or criminal. HPI does not separate the components of the domain classification such as the setting, staff, patient, and patient care intervention as seen in the JC taxonomy.

However, HPI has separate taxonomies depicting Individual Failure Modes and System Failure Modes. These taxonomies are analogous to the JC's *cause* classification. Components are comparable in each of the taxonomies. The JC human subclassification explores possible patient factors that may lead to adverse events. However, the HPI taxonomy of Individual Failure Modes mainly probes failures that practitioners may commit such as unformed skills, inadequate knowledge, fatigue, tunnel vision, recklessness or indifference and does not touch on patients' involvement in the event. As Buetow et al. explain, "it is easy to confuse human error with blame and to view patients … as incapable of error because they can be sick and tend to have reduced power in their interactions with clinicians and the health system."[13] However, patients can contribute to medical errors that can lead to the "breakdown in the clinician-patient relationship"[13]; assertion errors (behaviors that prevent patients from communicating effectively with providers), adherence errors (patient noncompliance with medications), or action errors (patients do not attend medical visits or refuse care) are examples of patient factors that could lead to adverse events. Rather than focus on patient roles in adverse events, HPI identifies organizational faults that influence human errors; "root causes of events nearly always are found as deficiencies in organizational systems."[14]

The HPI taxonomy does not have a special classification for prevention and mitigation as the JC taxonomy does to specifically address corrective actions or action plans to prevent the reoccurrence of the adverse event in the future. Organizations that utilize the HPI method must decide on the corrective actions when performing the root cause analyses.

Future Classification Systems

These taxonomies offer important methods of characterizing and understanding patient safety events, their causes, and their potential solutions. While it is vital that institutions utilize similar approaches to their own patient safety culture to allow for standardization, which breeds uniformity and collaboration, we must also understand that these taxonomies are proposed frameworks and that we can continue to improve upon this framework as we use it to fit each healthcare institution and environment. While some changes to this framework may make sense for one institution, it may not for another. Continuing to share ideas and committing to collaborate to improve the methods by which we assess patient safety in our healthcare institutions will only make healthcare safer. Demonstrating a commitment to open and honest communication (and keeping legal protections in place permitting us to do so) by continuing to share lessons learned and methods to improve patient safety will continue to have a positive impact on our patients.

References

1. Chantler C. The role and education of doctors in the delivery of healthcare. *The Lancet*. 1999;353(9159):1178–181.

2. Kram R. Critical incident reporting system in emergency medicine. *Current Opinion in Anaesthesiology*. 2008;21(2):240–244.

3. Chang A, Schyve P, Croteau R, O'Leary D, and Loeb J. The JCAHO patient safety event taxonomy: A standardized terminology and classification schema for near misses and adverse events. *International Journal for Quality in Health Care*. 2005;17(2):95–105.

4. Tackling patient safety taxonomy: A must for risk managers. *Journal of Healthcare Risk Management*. 2008;28(1):7–17. P.7.

5. Joyce P, Boaden R, andEsmail A. Managing risk: A taxonomy of error in health policy. *Health Care Analysis*. 2005;13:337–46. P.338.

6. Larizgoitia I, Bouesseau M-C, and Kelley E. WHO efforts to promote reporting of adverse events and global learning. *Journal of Public Health Research*. January 2013;2(3):168–74.p.170.

7. Chang A. The JCAHO patient safety event taxonomy: A standardized terminology and classification schema for near misses and adverse events. *International Journal for Quality in Health Care*. 2005;17:95–105. P. 97.

8. Brixey J, Johnson T, and Zhang J. Evaluating a medical error taxonomy. AMIA 2002 Annual Symposium Proceedings:71–5.p.71.

9. Elder NC, and Dovey SM. Classification of medical errors and preventable adverse events in primary care: A synthesis of the literature. *The Journal of Family Practice*. 2002;31:927–32.

10. Throop C and Stockmeier C. The HPI SEC and SSER patient safety measurement system for healthcare. *HPI White Paper Series*, 2016; 1–32.

11. Chang A. The JCAHO patient safety event taxonomy: A standardized terminology and classification schema for near misses and adverse events. *International Journal for Quality in Health Care*. 2005;17:95–105.

12. Throop C and Stockmeier C. The HPI SEC and SSER patient safety measurement system for healthcare. *HPI White Paper Series*, 2011; 1–34.

13. Buetow S, Kiata L, Liew T, Kenealy T, Dovey S, and Elwyn G. Patient error: A preliminary taxonomy. *The Annals of Family Medicine*. 2009;7(3):223–231.

14. Throop C and Stockmeier C. The HPI SEC and SSER patient safety measurement system for healthcare. *HPI White Paper Series*, 2011; 1–34. p. 4.

Chapter 9

Databases and Surgical Quality Improvement: Pooling Our Data

Manon Haché and Cindy B. Katz

Database research has become increasingly more utilized in medicine. The evolution of the medical record into an electronic format has allowed the development of much more comprehensive data sets that can be imported from available data and accessed at a later date in order to evaluate the quality of care of our patients. The amount of available data and the speed at which it can be accessed is unprecedented. Administrative and clinical databases are available to answer many varied and clinically relevant questions. Databases as a means of capturing adverse events was discussed in Chapter 5.

Administrative databases have the advantage of being readily available and relatively inexpensive. However, they lack any clinical detail that could be useful for risk analysis and risk adjustment. The large size of administrative databases may result in rare events being found to be statistically significant between groups that may be clinically insignificant. This may be somewhat mitigated by using a case control analysis.[1]

Databases are also being utilized as a way to apply objective criteria to evaluating quality of care. In recent years, there has been an increasing interest in developing quality measures in order to better quantify the quality of care that various physicians and healthcare systems provide and its effects on patient safety. Various quality measures can be utilized, including process measures and outcomes measures.

In recent years, several large databases related to perioperative care have emerged. Advantages to using these databases include:[2]

- Comparing risk indexes among different institutions
- Looking at relatively rare complications by pooling data from multiple sources
- Focusing efforts on patient-centered outcomes analysis. Multiple outcomes can be studied
- Producing multidisciplinary goals and data-driven recommendations for care
- Analyzing trends of care
- Performing many different analyses on the same dataset
- Having potentially better external validity when compared to randomized controlled trials (RCTs), that is, datasets are not subject to inclusion or exclusion criteria
- Low cost

Limitations of database research include:

- Data type availability. Databases tend to be established without a specific question to answer. The data collected may not perfectly match the question that one is trying to answer.
- Incomplete data submissions. Data capture may be variable from one institution to the next.

- Inaccuracy of recorded data
- Insufficient audits of the database
- Not submitting negative outcomes
- Reverse causality is not determined but mere trends in care or outcome may be noted.

Comparing RCTs to Database Research

RCTs are the gold standard for researching the effects of treatments. However, when looking for a rare effect, they can be nearly impossible to complete. These trials are often too costly, too long, and require multicenter participation. Trials cannot be powered for unknown side effects. Results may not always apply to "real life" as all situations are controlled in RCTs, potentially making the trial situation artificial.

Database research can require propensity score matching in an attempt to decrease the effects of all potentially identifiable confounding variables. Strong outcomes data can come from variations in care, when we can retrospectively look at different management strategies to see if patients had different outcomes.

Existing Databases

One example of an important database that demonstrated a change in anesthesia practice is the Pediatric Perioperative Cardiac Arrest (POCA) project. This voluntary registry recorded perioperative pediatric cardiac arrests from 1994 to 2005. Around the time of its inception, a closed claims analysis of pediatric cardiac arrests was unable to determine the mechanism primarily responsible for these cardiac arrests. Published in 2000,[3] a retrospective analysis of this registry led to a change in practice when it was recognized that the primary cause of pediatric anesthesia-related perioperative cardiac arrests was attributed to medications, primarily cardiac depression from the use of Halothane. After its initial findings were published, a reanalysis of the registry published in 2007[4] demonstrated that the primary cause of pediatric anesthesia-related cardiac arrest had changed and was attributed to cardiovascular causes (mostly hypovolemia from bleeding or hyperkalemia from massive transfusion) rather than medications.

Wake Up Safe is a patient safety organization (PSO) established in 2008 by the Society for Pediatric Anesthesia (SPA). Its goals are to improve pediatric perioperative care through quality improvement efforts. It aims to address issues in processes of care in order to improve the quality of care of pediatric patients. Through the implementation of safety analytics and quality improvement, it strives to make the perioperative period safer for all children. It has grown to include 38 institutions, which contribute demographic information about all cases cared for by a pediatric anesthesiologist in addition to deidentified serious adverse event details. Serious adverse events are described as those occurring within 24 hours of the end of anesthesia care, either causing harm or a significant escalation of care for the patient. These include the following events:

- Airway injuries
- Airway management difficulties
- Awareness
- Blood transfusion complications
- Cardiac arrest
- Cardiovascular support

- Musculocutaneous complications
- Equipment issues
- Eye injuries
- Malignant hyperthermia
- Medication events
- Nervous system injuries
- Operating room fire
- Other injuries
- Perioperative deaths
- Respiratory events
- Wrong-sided procedures

All medication events and wrong-side procedures are captured regardless of degree of harm or escalation of care. All submitted cases are analyzed by three members at each participating institution through a root cause analysis process. In order to improve the capture and uniformity of events submitted, Wake Up Safe has developed educational tools for the members from participating institutions.

It is hoped that over time, trends and causes of rare serious adverse events may be able to be identified, and processes leading to these adverse events can be modified to decrease the risk associated with the occurrence of adverse events.

Since the inception of this initiative, a few patient safety alerts regarding medication safety and warnings, including one on the risk of acetaminophen overdose, have been published by members of Wake Up Safe. The advent of intravenous acetaminophen combined with the fact that electronic medical records do not always interface with the anesthesia record make this area particularly at risk for communication failure. Wake Up Safe has also issued a statement regarding prevention of wrong-side surgery and decreasing the risk of hyperkalemia related to blood transfusion therapy.

Articles were published about the inception of the Wake Up Safe organization and its database,[5] and about the quality improvement methods utilized by different institutions. Other articles reporting serious safety events were published, with events including wrong-sided frenulectomy,[6] bupivacaine overdose,[7] and hyperkalemia following massive transfusion.[8] Articles utilizing the database have also been published detailing reported cardiac arrests,[9] a subset of those cardiac arrests occurring in the postanesthesia care unit,[10] and medication errors.[11]

The limitations of this database include its voluntary nature and its multicenter participation which may lead to different reporting practices.

The Society for Thoracic Surgery (STS) has established a national database that collects clinical information on patients undergoing adult cardiac, pediatric and congenital cardiac, and general thoracic surgery. The first database to be created was the Adult Cardiac database, and at this time, more than 90% of all Adult Cardiac Surgery Centers participate in the database. Since its inception in 1989, more than 5 million cases have been reported to the database and currently there are more than 3,000 participating physicians.[12] The goal of this voluntary reporting database is to guide quality improvement initiatives and to produce guidelines. Participants agree to voluntary public reporting and benchmarking against national performance standards including risk-adjusted performance outcomes.

Several quality performance measures are currently being evaluated by STS.[13]

Greater than 100 research projects have been published using this database reporting on many different complications, discharge status, and mortality. More recently, studies were published analyzing national trends in clinical practice. A recent review article detailed the various research projects published using the database.[14]

The American College of Surgeons (ACS) founded its own quality improvement program in 2004. The National Surgical Quality Improvement Program (NSQIP) is a validated, risk-adjusted, outcomes-based program to measure and improve the quality of surgical care. Benefits of participation include: "identifying quality improvement targets, improving patient care and outcomes, and decreasing institutional healthcare costs" (ACS NSQIP Pediatric January 2019 Semiannual Report). Surgical outcomes improve in hospitals that participate in the ACS NSQIP.[15, 16] Several hundred hospitals in the United States participate in ACS NSQIP. NSQIP utilizes clinical data from each patient's medical record including preoperative, intraoperative, and postoperative variables. Outcomes data are risk adjusted for medical condition complexity and clinical relevance. Surgical patients are followed for 30 days to capture complications that may occur during admission or after discharge from the hospital.

Hospitals utilize trained and certified Surgical Clinical Reviewers to abstract clinical data from medical records. Detailed manual chart review is performed for every selected case that meets strict inclusion criteria. Outcomes tracked for 30 days include mortality, pneumonia, sepsis, urinary tract infection, venous thromboembolism, unplanned operation, readmission, and surgical site infection. Data is reported back to participating hospitals every six months in a semiannual report (SAR). The SAR demonstrates individual hospital outcomes compared to the observed or expected outcomes of all the other participating sites.

With surgical specialty outcomes data in hand, hospitals can look at their own guidelines and processes for improvement and seek mentoring opportunities as high outliers. The intent of NSQIP is to act on the data, monitor interventions with the data, and improve the quality of surgical care.

The American Society for Anesthesiology (ASA) founded the Anesthesia Quality Institute (AQI) in 2008 with a goal to develop the National Anesthesia Clinical Outcomes Registry (NACOR).[17]

AQI is a patient safety organization that has established the largest database for quality improvement in the field of anesthesiology. It has led efforts for improvement in care through education and data quality feedback. Many databases require manual entry. This makes the data entry very time-consuming and costly. NACOR uses billing or administrative data and can accept data from Anesthesia Information Systems, which automatically exports data into the database. All deidentified data is loaded into NACOR by AQI technologists and is extensively reviewed both automatically and manually to identify missing or erroneously entered data.

NACOR provides participating providers with performance monitoring, performance gap analysis, patient outlier identification, targeted education, and peer-to-peer benchmarking.

There are several methodological issues with using large databases for comparative effectiveness research. The International Society for Pharmacoeconomics and Outcomes Research is a leading educational and scientific organization for health economics and outcomes research. They formed a task force in 2007 to establish Good Research Practices for Designing and Analyzing Retrospective Databases. Their recommendations were published in 2009[18, 19, 20] and include the following:

(1) Study populations must be relevant to the question that is being asked.
(2) The quality and validity of the data entered must be described.
(3) Data quality checks and data cleaning procedures must be addressed.
(4) Databases may pool data from different sources.
(5) Data must be linked in a way that the same variable is entered the same way in each database.

In the past, databases used for research may not have been set up for that purpose. For example, billing databases may be missing certain health attributes which may not have been required for billing. The research design has to take into consideration what data is available in the database and explain any design weakness that may be present. Inclusion and exclusion criteria should be clearly described. Definitions and criteria should be supported by the literature.

In conclusion, several administrative and clinical databases have been established that can be used to improve patient safety and outcomes in perioperative medicine. These will be particularly helpful in studying rare complications which arise in the perioperative setting. The limitations of using secondary databases are well described and should be taken into account when drawing conclusions. Nonetheless, membership of and participation in data registries can be a useful part of a hospital's QI work, allowing benchmarking against an aggregate of data from peer institutions. Participation in data registries will tend to improve that institution's efforts to identify and investigate their own QI cases.

References

1. Zhan C and Miller MR. Administrative data based patient safety research: A critical review. *Quality & Safety in Health Care*. 2003;12(Suppl 2):ii58–63.

2. Fleischut PM, Mazumdar M, and Memtsoudis SG. Perioperative database research: Possibilities and pitfalls. *British Journal of Anaesthesia*. 2013;111(4):532–534.

3. Morray JP, Geiduschek JM, Ramamoorthy C, et al. Anesthesia-related cardiac arrest in children: Initial findings of the Pediatric Perioperative Cardiac Arrest (POCA) Registry. *Anesthesiology*. 2000;93(1):6–14.

4. Bhananker SM, Ramamoorthy C, Geiduschek JM, et al. Anesthesia-related cardiac arrest in children: Update from the Pediatric Perioperative Cardiac Arrest Registry. *Anesthesia & Analgesia*. 2007;105(2):344–350.

5. Kurth CD, Tyler D, Heitmiller E, Tosone SR, Martin L, and Deshpande JK. National pediatric anesthesia safety quality improvement program in the United States. *Anesthesia & Analgesia*. 2014;119(1):112–121.

6. Rampersad S, Rossi MG, Yarnell C, and Uejima T. Wrong site frenulectomy in a child: A serious safety event. *Anesthesia & Analgesia*. 2014;119(1):141–144.

7. Buck D, Kreeger R, and Spaeth J. Case discussion and root cause analysis: Bupivacaine overdose in an infant leading to ventricular tachycardia. *Anesthesia & Analgesia*. 2014;119(1):137–140.

8. Lee AC, Reduque LL, Luban NL, Ness PM, Anton B, and Heitmiller ES. Transfusion-associated hyperkalemic cardiac arrest in pediatric patients receiving massive transfusion. *Transfusion*. 2014;54(1):244–254.

9. Christensen RE, Lee AC, Gowen MS, Rettiganti MR, Deshpande JK, and Morray JP. Pediatric perioperative cardiac arrest, death in the off hours: A report from wake up safe, the pediatric quality improvement initiative. *Anesthesia & Analgesia*. 2018;127(2):472–477.

10. Christensen RE, Haydar B, and Voepel-Lewis TD. Pediatric cardiopulmonary arrest in the postanesthesia care unit, rare but preventable: Analysis of data from

wake up safe, the pediatric anesthesia quality improvement initiative. *Anesthesia & Analgesia.* 2017;124(4):1231–1236.

11. Lobaugh LMY, Martin LD, Schleelein LE, Tyler DC, and Litman RS. Medication errors in pediatric anesthesia: A report from the Wake up Safe quality improvement initiative. *Anesthesia & Analgesia.* 2017;125(3):936–942.

12. Shahian DM, Jacobs JP, Edwards FH, et al. The society of thoracic surgeons national database. *Heart.* 2013;99(20):1494–1501.

13. www.sts.org/quality-safety/performance-measures (Accessed 7/13/22).

14. Thourani VH, Badhwar V, Shahian DM, et al. The society of thoracic surgeons adult cardiac surgery database: 2019 update on research. *Annals of Thoracic Surgery.* August 2019;108(2):334–342.

15. Hall BL, Hamilton BH, Richards K, Bilimoria KY, Cohen ME, and Ko CY. Does surgical quality improve in the American College of Surgeons National Surgical Quality Improvement Program: An evaluation of all participating hospitals. *Annals of Surgery.* 2009;250(3):363–376.

16. Cohen ME, Liu Y, Ko CY, and Hall BL. Improved surgical outcomes for ACS NSQIP hospitals over time: Evaluation of hospital cohorts with up to 8 years of participation. *Annals of Surgery.* 2016;263(2):267–273.

17. Liau A, Havidich JE, Onega T, and Dutton RP. The national anesthesia clinical outcomes registry. *Anesthesia & Analgesia.* 2015;121(6):1604–1610.

18. Berger ML, Mamdani M, Atkins D, and Johnson ML. Good research practices for comparative effectiveness research: Defining, reporting and interpreting nonrandomized studies of treatment effects using secondary data sources: The ISPOR good research practices for retrospective database analysis task force report – Part I. *Value Health.* 2009;12(8):1044–1052.

19. Cox E, Martin BC, Van Staa T, Garbe E, Siebert U, and Johnson ML. Good research practices for comparative effectiveness research: Approaches to mitigate bias and confounding in the design of nonrandomized studies of treatment effects using secondary data sources: The international society for pharmacoeconomics and outcomes research good research practices for retrospective database analysis task force report – Part II. *Value Health.* 2009;12(8):1053–1061.

20. Johnson ML, Crown W, Martin BC, Dormuth CR, and Siebert U. Good research practices for comparative effectiveness research: Analytic methods to improve causal inference from nonrandomized studies of treatment effects using secondary data sources: The ISPOR good research practices for retrospective database analysis task force report – Part III. *Value Health.* 2009;12(8):1062–1073.

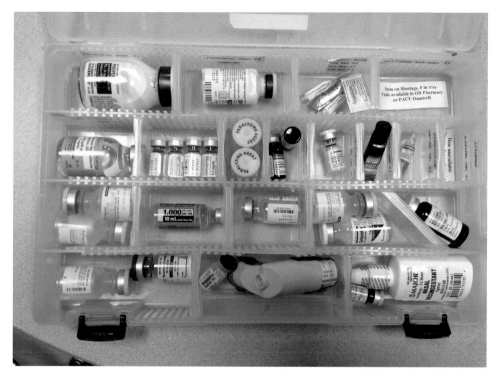

Figure 3.1 Original medication tray

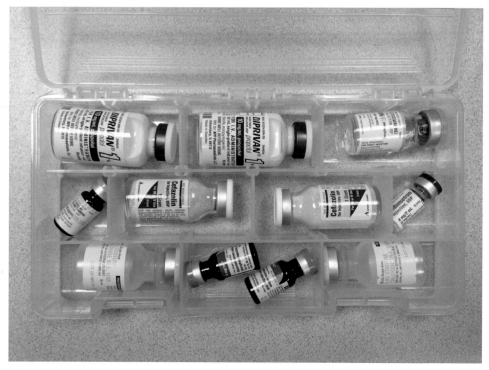

Figure 3.2 Primary medication tray

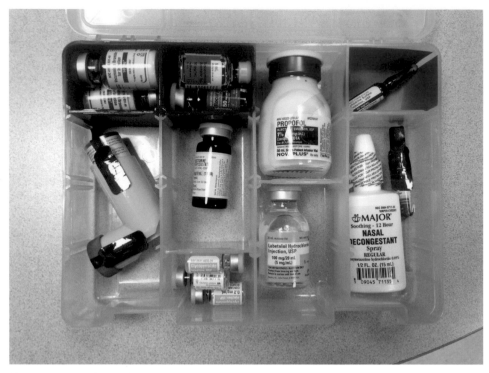

Figure 3.3 Secondary medication tray

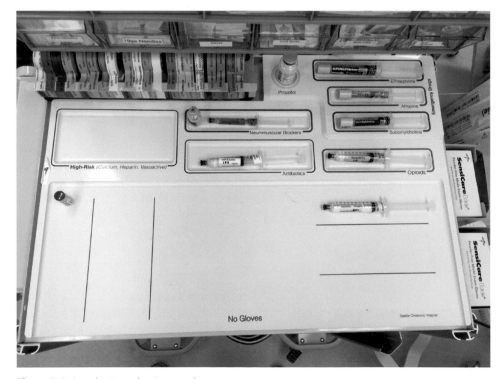

Figure 3.4 Anesthesia medication template

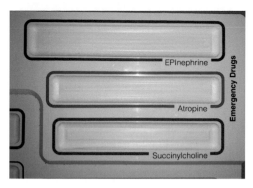

Figure 3.5 Color and background detail. *Original photos by Eliot Grigg and Figures 3.2 and 3.3 by Sally Rampersad; photos taken at Seattle Children's Hospital which did not require permission for their use.*

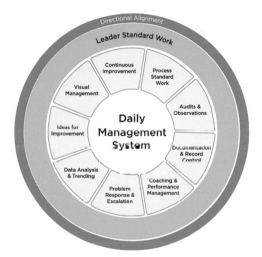

Figure 4.1 Daily management system. The DMS is a set of operational patterns practiced daily. Leader standard work envelops the routines, illustrating the importance of leadership routines to support an effective DMS.

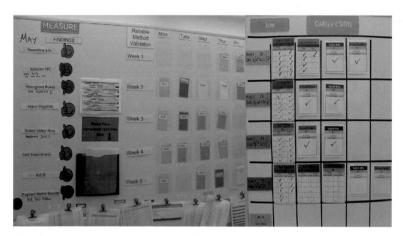

Figure 4.2 Standard work validation. This illustration provides two examples of a standard work validation method. Both examples communicate that the processes are part of the current validation, the status of the actual validation, and the results of observations.
Legends and figures supplied by Aaron Dipzinski, photos taken at Seattle Children's Hospital which did not require permission for their use.

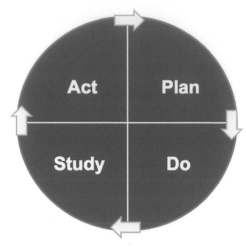

Figure 5.2 Plan-Do-Study-Act: CCC Rights Link permission obtained 6/10/21

Example KDD: Intraoperative Handoffs

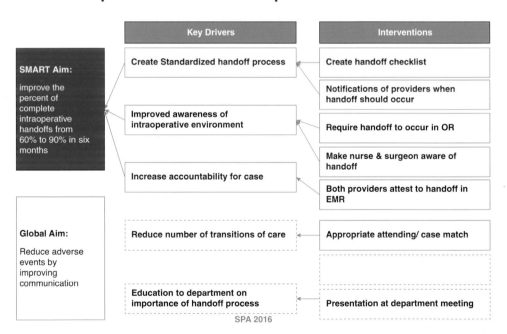

Figure 5.3 Key driver diagram: Permission obtained 6/10/21 IHI
Reprinted from www.IHI.org with permission of the Institute for Healthcare Improvement, ©2021.

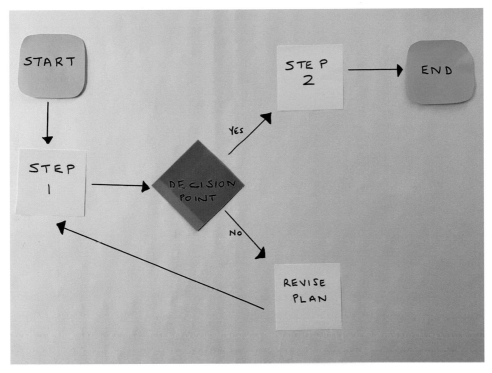

Figure 6.1 Process Map – original work of editor (SR), no permission needed

FISHBONE DIAGRAM

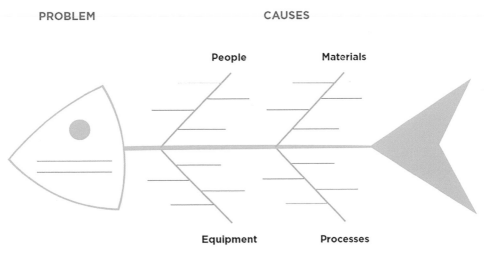

Figure 6.2 Fishbone – From SCH toolbox, no SCH logo, no permission needed

Anesthesia CQI

Please report ANY events you feel are important patient-safety events, even if it does not fit neatly into one of the categories listed below.

All medically important information should ALSO be documented in the legal medical record, as well as on this form.

Information in this REDCap form is privileged and confidential QI information. QI events are not legally discoverable under RCW 4.24.250 and 70.41.200.

Patient Name

Patient DOB

Patient MRN

Patient CSN

Name of reporter

Date of Service

Epic Log ID (please include if takeback / repeat case for patient on same date of service)

Describe Event

Cardiovascular
- ☐ Cardiac Arrest
- ☐ Chest Compressions
- ☐ Arrhythmia Requiring Treatment
- ☐ Unplanned Hypotension > 5 min Requiring Therapy
- ☐ Unplanned Hypertension> 5 min Requiring Therapy

Respiratory
- ☐ Hypoxia (without cyanotic CHD) > 60 sec
- ☐ Hypercapnia (ETCO2 > 70 mmHg)
- ☐ Bronchospasm Requiring Therapy
- ☐ Laryngospasm Requiring Pharmacologic Therapy
- ☐ Aspiration
- ☐ Pulmonary Edema
- ☐ Failed or Unanticipated Difficult Airway
- ☐ Unplanned Intubation or Reintubation in OR/PACU
- ☐ Unplanned Post-Operative Mechanical Ventilation

Trauma
- ☐ Dental or Facial Injury
- ☐ Other Injury

Describe trauma other injury

Pharmacologic
- ☐ Adverse Drug Reaction
- ☐ Incorrect Drug or Dose
- ☐ Medication Not Readily Available
- ☐ Transfusion Reaction
- ☐ Emergency Blood Transfusion
- ☐ Infusion or Pump-Related Error

Regional anesthesia complication
- ○ Yes
- ○ No

Miscellaneous
- ☐ Necessary Equipment Not Readily Available
- ☐ Equipment or Machine Failure
- ☐ Unplanned Case Delay
- ☐ Invasive Monitoring Complication
- ☐ Case Cancelled
- ☐ Other

Describe miscellaneous other

Figure 7.1 Reporting template – Anesthesia CQI blank from SCH, which did not require permission for its use

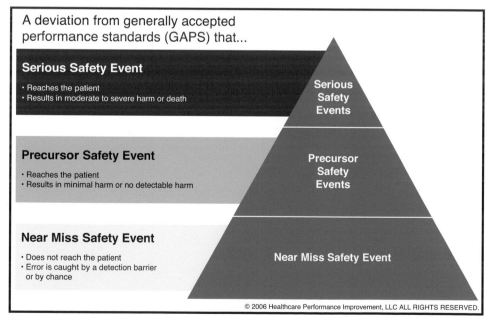

A deviation from generally accepted performance standards (GAPS) that...

Serious Safety Event
- Reaches the patient
- Results in moderate to severe harm or death

Serious Safety Events

Precursor Safety Event
- Reaches the patient
- Results in minimal harm or no detectable harm

Precursor Safety Events

Near Miss Safety Event
- Does not reach the patient
- Error is caught by a detection barrier or by chance

Near Miss Safety Event

Figure 8.1 HPI Structural Approach to Safety Events Classification. Reproduced with *permission from Press Ganey* "used with permission from Press Ganey Healthcare Performance Improvement (HPI). Copyright 2018"

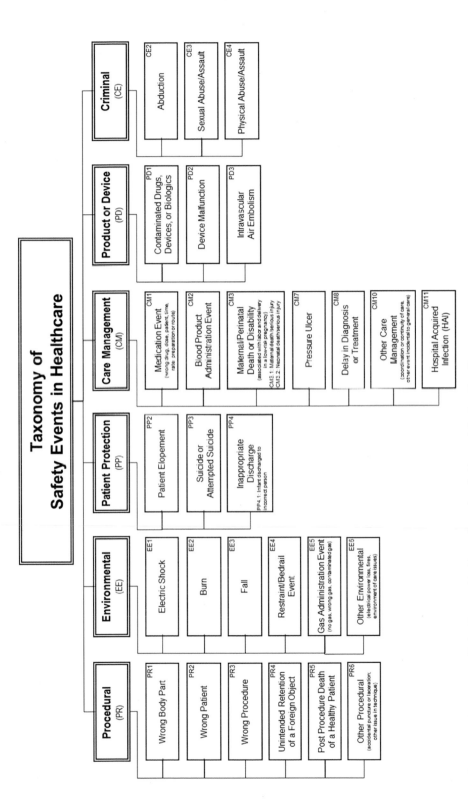

Figure 8.2 HPI Taxonomy of Safety Events in Healthcare. Reproduced with *permission from Press Ganey* "used with permission from Press Ganey Healthcare Performance Improvement (HPI). Copyright 2018."

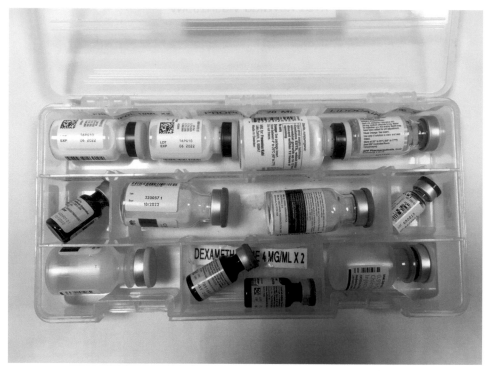

Figure 10.1 Medication trays

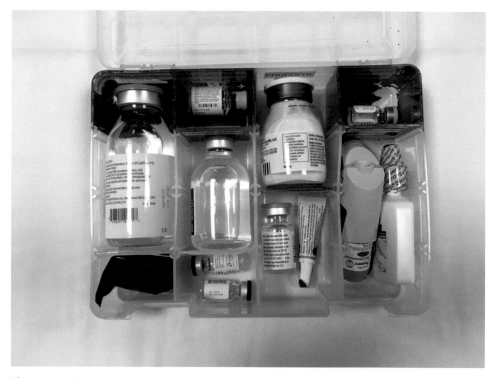

Figure 10.2 Cart top

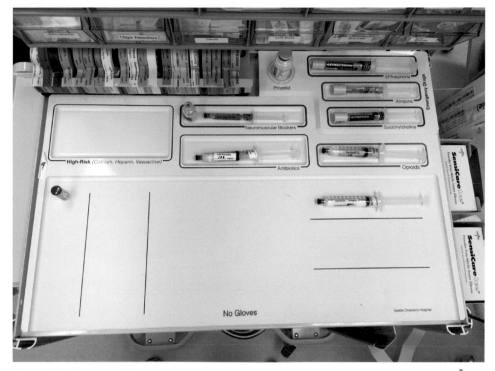

Figure 10.3 Medication labels

RISK Nurse Huddle Process

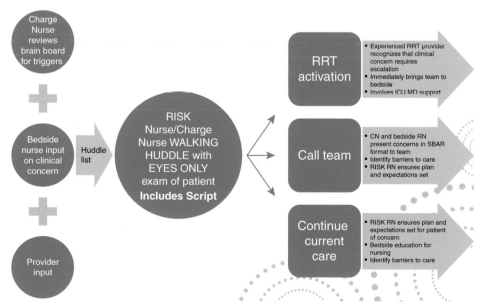

Figure 11.1 RISK RN huddle process

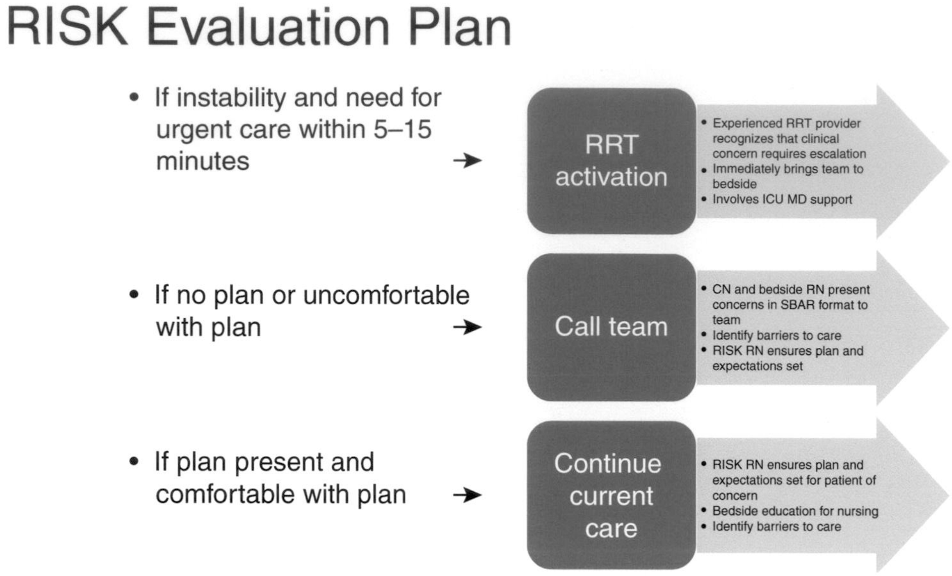

RISK Evaluation Plan

- If instability and need for urgent care within 5–15 minutes →

RRT activation
- Experienced RRT provider recognizes that clinical concern requires escalation
- Immediately brings team to bedside
- Involves ICU MD support

- If no plan or uncomfortable with plan →

Call team
- CN and bedside RN present concerns in SBAR format to team
- Identify barriers to care
- RISK RN ensures plan and expectations set

- If plan present and comfortable with plan →

Continue current care
- RISK RN ensures plan and expectations set for patient of concern
- Bedside education for nursing
- Identify barriers to care

Figure 11.2 RISK RN Evaluation

Day One

Time	Topic
07:00–07:10 hrs	Introductions
07:10–07:45 hrs	Overview of RISK Project • Background • Severe clinical deterioration definition • Daily work overview
07:45–08:45 hrs	Rapid Response • MPEWS Tool • Escalation Algorithm & RISK RN • Role and Responsibilities • Event Record
08:45–09:00 hrs	**Break**
09:00–10:00 hrs	Teamwork and Communication • Learn and understand how to use a structured communication technique to facilitate effective communication
10:00–11:00 hrs	Systematic Approach Algorithm • Why it is important • Systematic Approach Algorithm • Simulation/Practice
11:00–11:45 hrs	**Lunch**
11:45–13:00 hrs	Parent Prespective
13:00–14:00 hrs	RISK Huddles • Roles & Responsibilities • Surveillance Tool
14:00–14:15 hrs	**Break**
14:15–15:00 hrs	MPEWS Escalation Algorithm Pilot • Objectives • Algorithm review • Actions • Audit
15:00 hrs	Wrap up

Day Two

Time	Topic
07:00–11:00 hrs	**Simulation Scenarios**
11:00–12:00 hrs	**Break for Lunch**
12:00–15:00 hrs	**IV Training**

Figure 11.3 RISK RN Training

RISK RN Surveillance

Reason for RISK RN Evaluation

- ☑ RN/Provider/Parent concern
- ☐ RRT in last 24 hours
- ☐ Unfamiliar or off-pathway care
- ☐ MPEWS > = 5 in first 24 hours
- ☐ ED-ICU consult
- ☐ Other:

RISK RN Evaluation

Called to bedside for self limiting tachyarrythmias lasting only 30 seconds × 2. Patient sleeping and without complaint. Other vital signs and perfusion within normal range.

RISK RN Recommendation

- ○ Continue with current plan
- ◉ Notify team to clarify or modify plan (specify)
- ○ Call RRT & notify team to clarify/modify plan

Summary of Team Discussion

Team called to bedside to confirm ECG strip arrhythmias. 12 lead ECG performed. Team advised bedside RN to give lasix as ordered in the morning and will consider ordering lytes for am labs.

Communication Plan

- ☑ Primary contact MD/NP   ☑ RN
- ☑ Secondary contact MD/NP   ☑ Acute Care Charge nurse
- ☑ Attending
- ☑ Family
- ☑ ICU Charge nurse
- ☐ Respiratory Therapist

Recommended Update to Nursing Care Plan

Increases VS to q2h × 8hrs overnight. Include perfusion checks with VS and document in IView. Print ECG strips every shift and place in chart. If arrythmias occur, print strip and perform VS and perfusion check

Signs of deterioration to watch for

If hemodynamically unstable (low BP, CR >3sec, cool extremities, possibly altered LOC) call Code Blue. If tachyarrythmias occur again and hemodynamically stable (normal BP, CR <3sec, warm extremities) call cardiac transplant fellow and RRT.

RISK RN Actions

- ☑ Education
- ☐ IV start
- ☐ Suction patient
- ☐ Transport to Radiology
- ☐ Other:

Education Provided

- ☐ NP suction
- ☐ Fever management
- ☐ Airway positioning
- ☑ Signs/symptoms shock
- ☐ Signs/symptoms respiratory distress/failure
- ☐ Signs/symptoms increased ICP
- ☐ Other

Is Follow Up Needed?
- ○ No follow up needed
- ◉ Next follow up due

Next Follow Up Due 11/18/2013   0600

Figure 11.4 RISK RN surveillance form

MPEWS	UNIT	LOCATION	UNIT TM	PATIENT	MRN	AGE	SEX	ATTENDING P...	CONTACT PR...	ASSIGNED RN	ALERTS			RISK ALERTS		ALERT TM	STATUS
⊟ RRT Alerts (2)																	
	SUR-R6	RC.6.810-2	71:47	TEST, INSULIN TW...	5109270	19 Y	M	Lewin, Mark...	Morelli,S...					00:25 🔍 00:25		00:00	⊕ Add
12	CAN-F7	FA.7.219-1	3964:24	TESTING, SUCHIN...	5109043	3 Y	F	Gayer, Jeffre...	Morelli,S...					07:25 🔍 00:25		00:00	⊕ Add
⊟ MPEWS Alerts (1)																	
14	CAN-F8	FA.8.305-1	07:21	RISKRN, WENDY II	5109866	8 Y	F	McGuire, Tro...	Morelli, S...					14 00:25 🔍 00:25		00:00	⊕ Add
⊟ RISK Watch (1)																	
8 ↑	MED-R3	RB.3.420-2	1753:57	MONKEY, CEE	5108912	8 Y	M	Bull, Marta, P...	Morelli, S...		⚠	☆		🔍 00:25		00:00	⊕ Add
⊞ Completed Alerts (1)																	

Seattle Children's — RISK Safety Dashboard — As of 09/09/2013 @ 15:25 Help

Figure 11.5 RISK RN dashboard
All images created by the chapter authors, no permission required from Seattle Children's Hospital

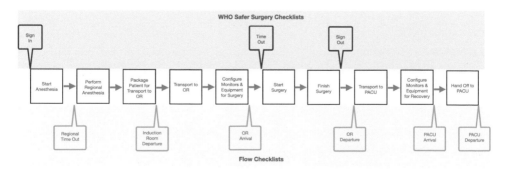

Figure 13.1 Patient Flow Checklist schematic indicating times when checklists are used

Regional Block Time-Out

Seattle Children's Main Operating Room

1. Anesthesiologist starts time-out
2. Starred (*) response first
3. RN initiates all other challenges
4. Emphasize all participants must verbally agree
5. If regional time-out is done simultaneously with surgical time-out, start with "block type" after surgical time-out is complete

6. Block site MUST be marked by the person performing the block. This can occur at any time, including during the time-out. Emphasize that the person marking should verify the location with a primary source such as consent. Bilateral and midline blocks do not need to be marked.

7. New local anesthetic dosing table

	Challenge	Regional Response	OR Anesthesia Response	RN Response
1 **AN**	Identify	Matches Consent	Matches CIS	**2** Reads Wrist Band
3 **RN**	Consent	Reads Consent		
	Surgical Site	Marked and Matches Consent	"Agree"	"Agree" **4**
	5 ··· START HERE IF COMBINING WITH SURGICAL TIME OUT ···			
	Block Type	States Block Type(s)		
	Block Site	Marks or Verifies Mark **6** At Block Sites(s)	"Correct"	"Correct"
RN	Allergies		Y/N and Specify	
	Skin Prep Restrictions		Y/N and Specify	
	Anticoagulation		Y/N and Specify **7**	
	Medication	State Medication Concentration (%), and Total Planned Dose (mL)	State Patient Weight	Verify Max Dose from Table
				View Drug Viat; Verify % and Expiration Date
		Draw up medication		
	Any Concerns?	**STATE CONCERN**		

Figures 13.2 Regional Timeout Checklist

Post-Handoff Checklist (v1.3)

Challenge	Who	Response
Manifold?	RN	Confirmed removed
Lines?	RN	Confirmed flushed
Oxygen Source Connected?	RN	Yes/Not Needed
Bed Sweep	Anesthesia	Inspect Bed
Orders?	Anesthesia	Yes/No
Good to Go?	Anesthesia	Yes/No

09/20

Figure 13.5 PACU Departure Checklist

	Maximum Dose Ropivacaine Plain OR Bupivacaine with Epinephrine 0.2% - 0.5% (3 mg/kg)		
Weight (kg)	0.2% (ml)	0.25% (mL)	0.5% (mL)
3	4	3	1
4	6	4	`2
5	7	6	3
6	9	7	3
7	10	8	4
8	12	9	4
9	13	10	5
10	15	12	6
12	18	14	7
14	21	16	8
16	24	19	9
18	27	21	10
20	30	24	12
22	33	26	13
24	36	28	14
26	39	31	15
28	42	33	16
30	45	36	18
32	48	38	19
34	51	40	20
36	54	43	21
38	57	45	22
40	60	48	24
42	63	50	25
44	66	52	26
46	69	55	27
48	72	57	28
50	75	60	30
52	78	62	31
54	81	64	32
56	84	67	33
58	87	69	34
60	90	72	36
>60	1.5 mL/kg	1.2 mL/kg	0.6 mL/kg
Note: Maximum Dose for Bupivacaine Plain is 2.5 mg/kg: 1 mL/kg (0.25%) or 0.5 mL/kg (0.5%)			

Figure 13.3 Regional Anesthesia Reference Dosing Table

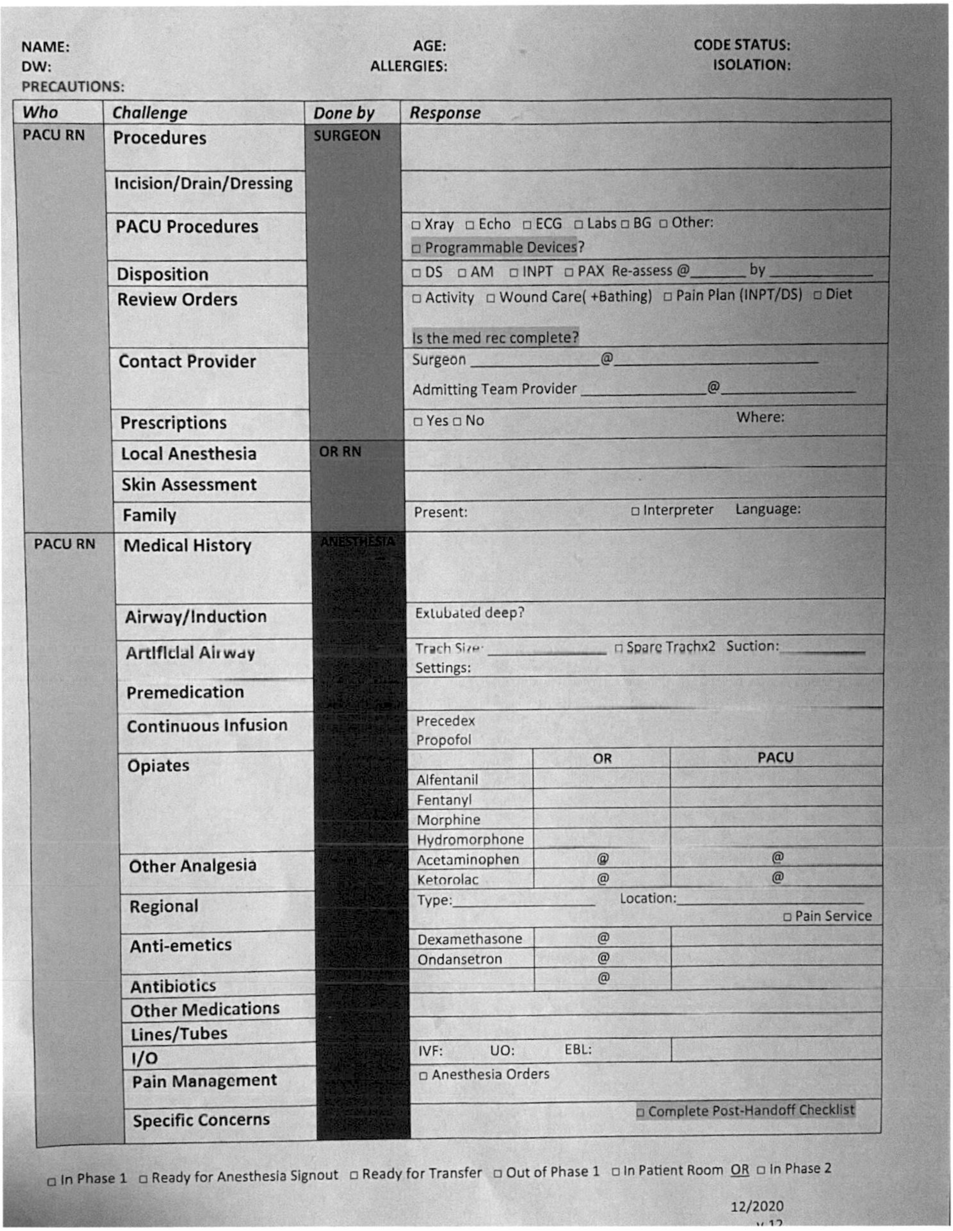

NAME:	AGE:	CODE STATUS:
DW:	ALLERGIES:	ISOLATION:
PRECAUTIONS:		

Who	Challenge	Done by	Response
PACU RN	Procedures	SURGEON	
	Incision/Drain/Dressing		
	PACU Procedures		□ Xray □ Echo □ ECG □ Labs □ BG □ Other: □ Programmable Devices?
	Disposition		□ DS □ AM □ INPT □ PAX Re-assess @_____ by _____
	Review Orders		□ Activity □ Wound Care(+Bathing) □ Pain Plan (INPT/DS) □ Diet Is the med rec complete?
	Contact Provider		Surgeon _____ @_____ Admitting Team Provider _____ @_____
	Prescriptions		□ Yes □ No Where:
	Local Anesthesia	OR RN	
	Skin Assessment		
	Family		Present: □ Interpreter Language:
PACU RN	Medical History	ANESTHESIA	
	Airway/Induction		Extubated deep?
	Artificial Airway		Trach Size:_____ □ Spare Trachx2 Suction:_____ Settings:
	Premedication		
	Continuous Infusion		Precedex Propofol
	Opiates		

			OR	PACU
	Opiates		Alfentanil	
			Fentanyl	
			Morphine	
			Hydromorphone	
	Other Analgesia		Acetaminophen @	@
			Ketorolac @	@
	Regional		Type:_____ Location:_____ □ Pain Service	
	Anti-emetics		Dexamethasone @	
			Ondansetron @	
	Antibiotics		@	
	Other Medications			
	Lines/Tubes			
	I/O		IVF: UO: EBL:	
	Pain Management		□ Anesthesia Orders	
	Specific Concerns		□ Complete Post-Handoff Checklist	

□ In Phase 1   □ Ready for Anesthesia Signout   □ Ready for Transfer   □ Out of Phase 1   □ In Patient Room OR □ In Phase 2

12/2020
v.12

Figure 13.4 PACU Handoff Checklist

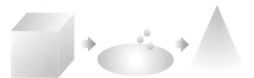

Figure 15.1 Lewin's freeze/unfreeze Model
Reproduced with permission from Mind Tools

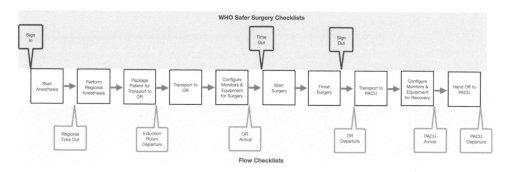

Figure 15.3 Checklist workflow (created by the author, SCH did not require permission for use)

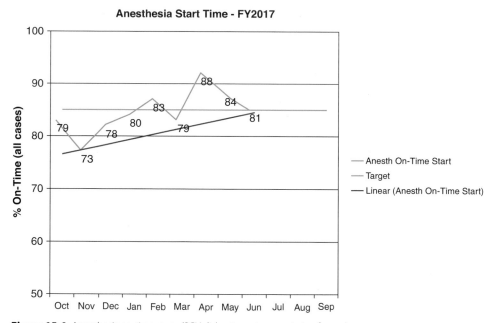

Figure 15.4 Anesthesia on-time starts (SCH did not require permission for use)

Chapter

10

Medication Safety at a Pediatric Hospital and Failure Modes Effects Analysis: A Series of Projects Undertaken to Address the Issue of Medication Errors in the Operating Room

Lizabeth D. Martin

A failure mode and effects analysis (FMEA) is a validated systematic improvement methodology to prospectively evaluate risk and guide targeted interventions. It was developed by the United States military and has been utilized in aviation, the nuclear industry, and increasingly in healthcare.[1, 2, 3] This step-by-step approach involves analyzing a process, in this case medication handling, by deconstructing it into multiple discrete steps. For every process step, potential failures are identified and prioritized according to how serious their consequences are, how frequently they occur, and how easily they can be detected. The process differs from commonly utilized retrospective improvement methodologies, such as Root Cause Analyses, which are used to investigate safety events after they occur.[4, 5, 6]

Medication errors are an important cause of preventable harm and continue to draw attention from regulators, institutions, providers, and consumers.[7] In anesthesia practice, medication errors have proven difficult to study; the literature is largely limited to retrospective or self-reported data, and specific processes to reduce intraoperative medication errors are lacking.[8, 9, 10, 11] There are unique aspects of medication handling in the operating room that incur risk. Anesthesiologists are the only healthcare providers who independently perform all steps in the medication handling process: prescribing, preparing, administering, monitoring, and recording. High-risk medications are given in an environment with many potential distractions. This often occurs without added safety mechanisms such as computer decision support, pharmacy review, or independent double checks, which are standard in other healthcare arenas. Pediatric anesthesia practice, in particular, may create additional risks because of the increased need for dilution and manipulation of medications and weight-based dosing calculations without formal cognitive support.[12, 13, 14] Although many of these errors may not directly translate to patient harm, some can lead to devastating consequences.[15, 16]

The objectives of this quality improvement project were to systematically deconstruct the intraoperative medication handling process by pediatric anesthesiologists at our institution; identify and quantify areas of risk; implement a bundle of targeted countermeasures; and collect medication error data before, during, and after implementation. We describe five specific projects addressing medication errors in the operating room that were generated through this process.

Developing the Interventions

Literature review: What is the evidence?

First, a comprehensive literature review was conducted to understand the scope of the problem and the solutions that have been proposed and to establish evidence supporting specific interventions. Evidence-based recommendations for medication safety in the operating room include the standardization of medication organization in the anesthesia workspace, formal organization of vials and syringes to minimize swaps, syringe labeling, use of prefilled or pharmacy-prepared syringes, inventory management, and development of robust error-reporting systems.[13, 17, 18, 19, 20] Trends in operating room medication safety encourage shifting the burden of responsibility from individual providers "being more careful" to system modifications that will achieve higher levels of error proofing.

Observations

A multidisciplinary team was formed, consisting of anesthesiologists, pharmacists, nurses, and a process improvement consultant. All team members conducted direct observations of the medication-handling process, including administration errors, syringe labeling, infusion checks, and handoff practices by anesthesia providers. This took place in the operating room over a two-month period using a standard audit tool, which was developed based on previously published medication error definitions, QI data, and nationally accepted best practice recommendations.[17, 19, 21, 22] After a total of 133 hours of observations, the team met over three days to systematically deconstruct and evaluate each step in the anesthesia medication handling process and identify risk using an FMEA. Nineteen process steps were identified in an anesthesia provider's workflow prescribing, preparing, dispensing, administering, monitoring, and recording medications, and one to eight possible "failure modes" were identified by the team for each process step. Each possible failure mode was then scored and ranked based on severity in the event of failure, occurrence rate, and ease of detection. The risk priority number (RPN) was calculated by multiplying severity × occurrence × detection. Failure modes with the highest RPN were considered for targeted intervention.[23, 24]

Interventions

Three high-risk categories were identified: (1) nonstandard organization of medications in the anesthesia work area; (2) syringe preparation: nonstandard syringe sizes, nonstandard medication dilutions, and suboptimal labeling practices; and (3) lack of double-check processes for medication infusions. The following five projects were identified and tested with repeated Plan-Do-Check-Act improvement cycles:

(1) Medication tray reorganization: medication vials are dispensed to anesthesiologists in pharmacy-prepared medication trays. The team observed disorganized medication vial dispensing. The original medication tray was redesigned into two separate trays to minimize the risk of vial swap and inadvertent administration of high-risk medications like vasopressors and muscle relaxants (Figure 10.1). Design principles that were used included sequestering and color-coding drugs with the highest harm potential, physical separation of look-alike and sound-alike vials, and simplification of the available medications. These design principles are discussed

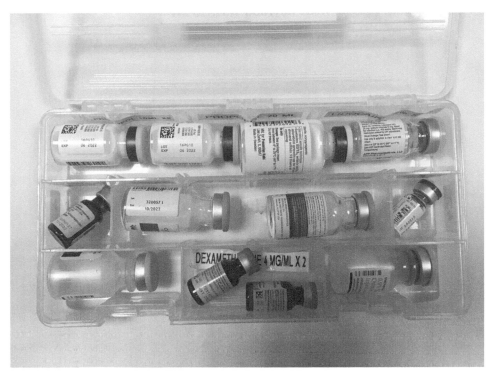

Figure 10.1 Medication trays
(A black and white version of this figure will appear in some formats. For the color version, refer to the plate section.)

in more detail in Chapter 3. The primary tray includes frequently used medications (i.e., propofol, ondansetron, dexamethasone, cefazolin). The secondary tray includes higher risk medications (i.e., muscle relaxants, vasopressors, reversal agents), and infrequently used medications (albuterol, oxymetazoline, dextrose), which anesthesia providers intentionally choose to access as needed.

(2) Medication cart top template: the team observed that there was no consistent organization or location for common medications in the anesthesia workspace. The medication cart top template was designed to standardize the organization of medication syringes. Human factors and design experts at the University of Washington School of Design collaborated with anesthesiologists to create a functional standard template to minimize the risk of syringe swaps. Designating a location for emergency medications on the anesthesia cart standardizes placement of these critical medications across all operating rooms and provides a visual cue to the anesthesia team if syringes are not present (Figure 10.2). These design principles are also discussed further in Chapter 3.

(3) Syringe labeling: medication labels with standard nomenclature and color-coding were ordered for all commonly used intraoperative medications. The anesthesia carts were modified to allow large tape dispensers to provide easy access to drug labels and thus safe syringe labeling practices. Emergency medications (succinylcholine, atropine, and epinephrine) were dispensed in standardized prefilled PharMEDium® medication syringes, ensuring standard concentration, syringe size, and labeling in all operating rooms (Figure 10.3).

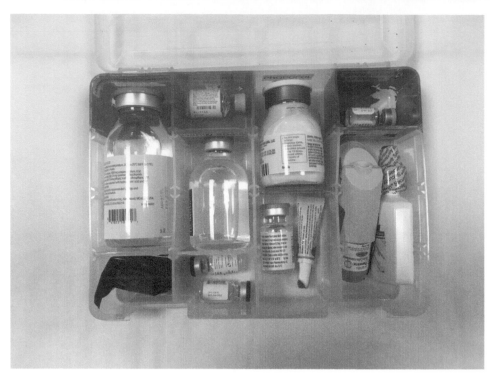

Figure 10.2 Cart top
(A black and white version of this figure will appear in some formats. For the color version, refer to the plate section.)

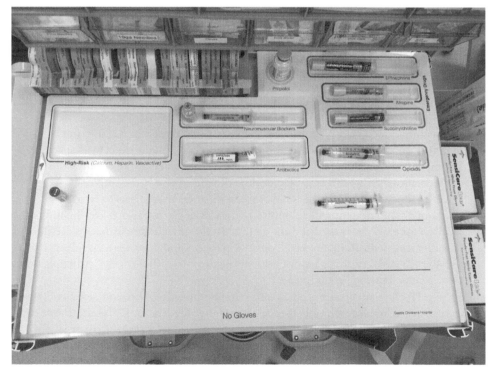

Figure 10.3 Medication labels
(A black and white version of this figure will appear in some formats. For the color version, refer to the plate section.)

(4) Infusion double check: A standard independent two-provider check process for infusions was developed based on institutionally accepted nursing double-check practice for confirming the "5 Rights" (right patient, medication, dose, route, and time) of medication administration. In addition, the unique aspects of anesthesia work flow (fast paced, sole anesthesia provider, infusion pump variation) were considered, and a process was developed that could be applied to infusion types ranging from propofol in rapid turnover rooms to epidural or peripheral nerve catheter infusions. An "infusion checked" labeling tape applied to the tubing provides a visual cue that a double check has been performed. The two-provider check evolved through 14 iterations of the process of trialing, provider feedback, and implementation.

(5) A medication practice guideline was developed and posted in every operating room. This included syringe labeling and preparation expectations, standard syringe sizes and dilution recommendations, and modification of the preprocedural regional block "time out" to include a weight-based maximum local anesthetic dose calculation with a laminated job aid prior to local anesthetic preparation.

Implementation

The implementation phase incorporated trialing, feedback, and tests of change for each of the countermeasures described above.

Implementation strategies for the interventions that involved physical changes in the anesthesia work-space (medication trays, cart top template) involved well-defined test sequences. First, the design was vetted with the team and subsequently with anesthesiologists from multiple clinical areas. Feedback was collected and incorporated by team members via face-to-face demonstration as well as formal (written) survey tools. Anesthesia providers were educated about the new practice guidelines by presentation and question and answer sessions at a departmental meeting, electronic newsletter, and poster displays immediately prior to implementation. A follow-up survey tool was performed, and minor adjustments based on provider feedback continued after initial implementation for each countermeasure.

Incorporation of the infusion checklist required a change in the workflow of anesthesia providers and thus required a different trialing and implementation process. First, the checklist was trialed by team members in various clinical work areas (GI suite, interventional radiology, cardiac room), with various infusion types to ensure the check would be applicable to all workflows. Through a series of 14 iterations of trialing and feedback, the final version was created. All anesthesia providers were educated on the infusion checklist guideline by a presentation at a staff meeting, an announcement in the weekly newsletter, and electronic reminders the week before implementation. In addition, each member of the anesthesia department was individually educated on how to perform the infusion check by a member of the medication safety team. Questions were answered and best practices shared during these one-on-one sessions. Team members provided coaching and feedback to providers for three weeks after implementation.

To sustain the interventions, expectations of the five countermeasures above are incorporated into regular orientation for rotating residents, fellows, and new faculty members.

Results

Process measures and outcomes were defined to measure the impact of the interventions. Process measures included syringe labeling, cart top organization, and two-provider check compliance and were audited before and after the interventions. Outcomes included medication errors, reported as the average number of errors per 1,000 anesthetics, and near-miss medication errors, defined as errors that were identified but did not reach the patient. Data from preexisting hospital and departmental QI reporting mechanisms were tabulated before, during, and after implementation of these projects. In addition, an anonymous error reporting system with biweekly reminders to all anesthesia providers was developed to encourage error reporting, including near-miss situations.

Process Measures

Preimplementation audit data were collected using a standard audit tool by multidisciplinary team members for 133 hours during 68 cases. A total of 368 prepared syringes were audited and 101 labeling errors were identified. There was no standard organization for medications in the anesthesia workspace in this preimplementation phase. Infusion pumps were double-checked in 4/17 (23%) cases and were not double-checked in the remainder of cases; double checks that were performed were conducted in a random manner because a standard process did not yet exist.

Postimplementation audit data for 61 randomly selected cases over a two-month period were collected using a standard audit tool. A total of 402 medication syringes were audited, and 16 labeling errors (4.0%) were identified. The medication cart top template was located on all anesthesia carts. Emergency medications (succinylcholine, atropine, and epinephrine PharMEDium® prefilled syringes) were located in the assigned standard location in standard syringes in 100% of cases. Other medications were located in their designated location in 78/97 (80%) instances (muscle relaxants 81%, opioids 74%, antibiotics 90%, and high-risk medications 71%). A two-provider check was performed in 10/17 (59%) cases with medication infusions.

Outcomes

Preimplementation, a historic baseline of 0.12 medication errors were reported per 1,000 anesthetics. Anonymous error reporting mechanisms were introduced, and self-reported medication errors increased to a median error rate of 1.56 errors per 1,000 anesthetics, which established the preimplementation error rate for subsequent comparisons. Near-miss event reporting increased from 0 to 1.3 per month after the introduction of anonymous error reporting. The countermeasures were subsequently implemented, and data collection continued. Postimplementation, medication errors decreased to an average of 0.95 errors per 1,000 anesthetics with continued consistent reporting of near-miss events at an unchanged rate compared to preimplementation. A run chart describing medication error rates per 1,000 anesthetics over time demonstrated a significant decrease in error rates with 18 consecutive points below the median since countermeasure implementation (Figure 10.4). The frequency of medication error harm events (NCC MERP E-I Harm events as above) has decreased since implementation (countermeasures implemented between August 2013 and August 2014), with nine harm events in 2013, five in 2014, and

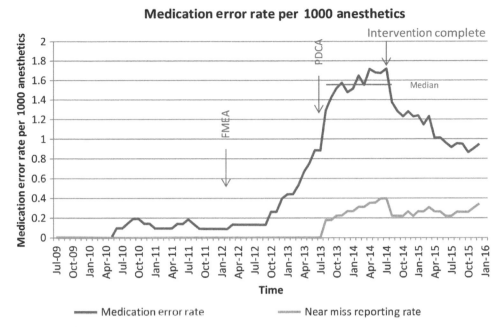

Figure 10.4 Total medication error rates from 2010 to 2016, reported as medication errors per 1,000 anesthetics averaged over 12 prior months

four in 2015. There were 10 infusion pump or delivery errors reported preintervention. Of the ten errors reported postimplementation, four near-miss events were caught by the check process before reaching the patient. After implementation, a decrease in swap, prescribing, preparation, and miscalculation errors was reported.

Analysis

Run charts are commonly used to display QI data and can be used to systematically determine whether the process is displaying a nonrandom pattern. For a run chart, statistically significant change occurs when six consecutive points are all above or below the median centerline, or five consecutive points are all increasing or decreasing.[19] Medication errors per 1,000 anesthetic cases were charted on a run chart to follow error rates over time before, during, and after the intervention.

Discussion

This chapter describes the implementation of five target interventions that were designed through systematically evaluating the medication handling processes of anesthesiologists. Direct observational data showing an improvement in best practice process measures (syringe labeling, workspace standardization, and double checks), as well as trends in decreasing medication errors, suggest that this process can be successfully utilized to improve safety in the operating room.

Challenges were encountered with implementation of the described changes. Making well-vetted modifications to the anesthesia workspace (medication trays, cart top template) was relatively straightforward to implement and well received by providers. However, inspiring a change that increased the workload of anesthesiologists (e.g., two-provider infusion check) has proven more challenging to implement, with incomplete success. As such, compliance with two-provider checks of infusion pumps only improved from 23% (using a nonstandard double-check process) to 59% (standardized double-check procedure). Although four pump programming errors were successfully caught postintervention, some errors still reached the patient, which is likely due to noncompliance with the standard process. This process was more successfully implemented in small teams (regional anesthesia and cardiac anesthesia teams) compared to the general operating room.

Limitations

The medication error data presented is predominately self-reported, which tends to underestimate actual error rates.[30] Well-recognized challenges to capturing accurate medication error data include embarrassment, fear of legal or disciplinary processes, additional work, fatigue, or normalization of deviance.[31, 32] In an attempt to address this limitation, the authors incorporated an anonymous error reporting system, regular email reminders, and orientation education for rotating trainees and faculty.

Although medication error self-reporting has improved at our institution, reported error rates (1.56/1,000 anesthetics) remain much lower than those reported with prospective observational data (84 errors/1,000 anesthetics at our institution or 552 errors/1,000 anesthetics at others[33]). Thus, it is likely that errors continue to be underreported. The observed decrease in medication error rates postintervention that we describe could be attributable to reporting fatigue – a decrease in error reporting over time rather than an actual decrease in medication errors. The sustained reporting of near-miss errors, errors that have the potential to cause harm but do not reach the patient, suggests that reporting was sustained throughout the auditing period. Regular reminders via email and departmental meetings have continued to optimize reporting.

Conclusions

Medication errors are an important problem in the practice of anesthesiology. They have historically been underreported, can be challenging to identify, and have proven difficult to study with traditional scientific methodology. For this reason, a multidisciplinary team elected prospectively to identify areas of risk systematically using an FMEA. Although standardization, labeling, and syringe sizes may help to mitigate dosing errors, these interventions do not directly address dose calculation, which is routinely required for precise weight-based dosing in pediatric anesthesia practice. Technology such as bar coding may have promising potential, and it is anticipated that ongoing investigation in this area will demonstrate a safety benefit that justifies cost and will provide further guidance for incorporating these practices reliably into anesthesia workflow.[10, 20, 34, 35] Even with the hopeful future implementation of improved technology, it is unlikely that there will be a single "silver bullet" solution that addresses many potential failure modes in the complex perioperative setting. More likely, true progress will come from a comprehensive evaluation of the entire medication handling system, and a bundle of interventions will be necessary, including standardization, education, a safety culture, and institution-specific interventions based on reported errors through QI processes. This project incorporates best practice recommendations into a bundle of low-cost, simple, usable interventions designed by anesthesiologists that have improved medication safety at one institution.

References

1. Cheng CH, Chou CJ, Wang PC, et al. Applying HFMEA to prevent chemotherapy errors. *Journal of Medical Systems.* 2012;36(3):1543–1551.

2. van Tilburg CM, Leistikow IP, Rademaker CM, et al. Health care failure mode and effect analysis: A useful proactive risk analysis in a pediatric oncology ward. *Quality and Safety in Health Care.* 2006;15(1):58–63.

3. Rosen MA, Sampson JB, Jackson EV, Jr., et al. Failure mode and effects analysis of the universal anaesthesia machine in two tertiary care hospitals in Sierra Leone. *British Journal of Anaesthesia.* 2014;113(3):410–415.

4. Chang DS, Chung JH, Sun KL, et al. A novel approach for evaluating the risk of health care failure modes. *Journal of Medical Systems.* 2012;36(6):3967–3974.

5. DeRosier J, Stalhandske E, Bagian JP, et al. Using health care failure mode and effect analysis: The VA National Center for patient safety's prospective risk analysis system. *Joint Commission Journal on Quality and Patient Safety.* 2002;28(5):248–267, 209.

6. Chatman I, ed., *Failure Mode and Effects Analysis in Health Care: Proactive Risk Reduction.* Oakbrook, IL, The Joint Commission, 2010.

7. Institute of Medicine CoQHCiA. *To Err Is Human, Building a Safer Health System.* Washington, D.C., Report of the Institute of Medicine, 2000.

8. Abeysekera A, Bergman IJ, Kluger MT, and Short TG. Drug error in anaesthetic practice: A review of 896 reports from the Australian Incident Monitoring Study database. *Anaesthesia.* 2005;60(3):220–227.

9. Llewellyn RL, Gordon PC, Wheatcroft D, Lines D, Reed A, Butt AD, et al. Drug administration errors: A prospective survey from three South African teaching hospitals. *Anaesthesia and Intensive Care.* 2009;37(1):93–98.

10. Orser BA, U D, and Cohen MR. Perioperative medication errors: building safer systems. *Anesthesiology.* 2016;124(1):1–3.

11. Tyler D. A Wake Up Safe Patient Safety Alert, Decreasing the Risks of Intravenous Medication Errors. *Wake Up Safe* 2010. Available at https://wakeupsafe.org/safety_alerts/157/ (Accessed 7/24/22).

12. Conroy S, Sweis D, Planner C, Yeung V, Collier J, Haines L, et al. Interventions to reduce dosing errors in children: A Systematic review of the literature. *Drug Safety.* 2007;30(12):1111–1125.

13. Merry AF and Anderson BJ. Medication errors – New approaches to prevention. *Paediatric Anaesthesia.* 2011;21(7):743–753.

14. Stucky ER. Prevention of medication errors in the pediatric inpatient setting. *Pediatrics.* 2003;112(2):431–436.

15. Cote CJ, Karl HW, Notterman DA, Weinberg JA, and McCloskey C. Adverse sedation events in pediatrics: Analysis of medications used for sedation. *Pediatrics.* 2000;106(4):633–644.

16. Paix AD, Bullock MF, Runciman WB, and Williamson JA. Crisis management during anaesthesia: Problems associated with drug administration during anaesthesia. *Quality and Safety in Health Care.* 2005;14(3):e15.

17. Eichhorn J. ASPF Hosts Medication Safety Conference, Consensus Group Defines Challenges and Opportunities for Improved Practice. [updated Spring 2010; cited 2016 December]. 1,3–8]. Available from: http://apsf.org/newsletters/html/2010/spring/index.htm (Accessed 10/14/2020).

18. ISMP. Key Vulnerabilities in the Surgical Environment: Container Mix-Ups and Syringe Swaps 2015 [cited 2016 December]. Available from: www.ismp.org/newsletters/acutecare/showarticle.aspx?id=123 (Accessed 10/14/2020).

19. Jensen LS, Merry AF, Webster CS, Weller J, Larsson L. Evidence-based strategies for preventing drug administration errors during anaesthesia. *Anaesthesia.* 2004;59(5):493–504.

20. Merry AF, Webster CS, Hannam J, Mitchell SJ, Henderson R, Reid P, et al. Multimodal system designed to reduce errors in recording and administration of drugs in anaesthesia: Prospective randomised clinical evaluation. *BMJ.* 2011;343:d5543.

21. ISMP. ISMP's list of High-Alert Medications 2012. Available from: www.ismp.org.**

22. Snyder RA, Abarca J, Meza JL, Rothschild JM, Rizos A, and Bates DW. Reliability Evaluation of the Adapted National Coordinating Council Medication Error Reporting and Prevention (NCC MERP) index. *Pharmacoepidemiology Drug Safety.* 2007;16(9):1006–1013.

23. Chatman I, ed. *Failure Mode and Effects Analysis in Health Care: Proactive Risk Reduction.* 3rd ed., Oakbrook, IL, The Joint Commission, 2010.

24. DeRosier J, Stalhandske E, Bagian JP, and Nudell T. Using health care failure mode and effect analysis: The VA National Center for patient safety's prospective risk analysis system. *Joint Commission Journal Quality Improvement.* 2002;28(5):248–267, 09.

25. Perla RJ, Provost LP, and Murray SK. The run chart: A simple analytical tool for learning from variation in healthcare processes. *BMJ Quality and Safety.* 2011;20(1):46–51.

26. Byrne AJ, Oliver M, Bodger O, Barnett WA, Williams D, Jones H, et al. Novel method of measuring the mental workload of anaesthetists during clinical practice. *British Journal of Anaesthesia.* 2010;105(6):767–771.

27. Ross V, Jongen EM, Wang W, Brijs T, Brijs K, Ruiter RA, et al. Investigating the influence of working memory capacity when driving behavior is combined with cognitive load: An LCT study of young novice drivers. *Accident Analysis Prevention.* 2014;62:377–387.

28. Grigg E, Martin LD, Ross F, Roesler A, Rampersad S, Haberkern C, Low D, Carlin K, Martin L. Assessing the impact of the anesthesia medication template on medication errors during anesthesia: A prospective study. *Anesthesia and Analgesia.* May 2017;124(5):1617–1625.

29. Yang Y, Rivera AJ, Fortier CR, and Abernathy JH, 3rd. A human factors engineering study of the medication delivery process during an anesthetic: Self-filled syringes versus prefilled syringes. *Anesthesiology.* 2016;124(4): 795–803.

30. Flynn EA, Barker KN, Pepper GA, Bates DW, and Mikeal RL. Comparison of methods for detecting medication errors in 36 hospitals and skilled-nursing facilities. *American Journal of Health System Pharmacy.* 2002;59(5):436–446.

31. Runciman B, Merry A, and Smith AM. Improving patients' safety by gathering information. Anonymous reporting has an important role. *BMJ.* 2001;323(7308):298.

32. Banja J. The normalization of deviance in healthcare delivery. *Business Horizons.* 2010;53(2):139.

33. Nanji KC, Patel A, Shaikh S, Seger DL, and Bates DW. Evaluation of perioperative medication errors and adverse drug events. *Anesthesiology.* 2016;124(1):25–34.

34. Jelacic S, Bowdle A, Nair BG, Kusulos D, Bower L, and Togashi K. A system for anesthesia drug administration using barcode technology: The Codonics safe label system and smart anesthesia manager. *Anesthesia and Analgesia.* 2015;121(2):410–421.

35. Webster CS, Larsson L, Frampton CM, Weller J, McKenzie A, Cumin D, et al. Clinical assessment of a new anaesthetic Drug Administration System: A prospective, controlled, longitudinal incident monitoring study. *Anaesthesia.* 2010;65(5):490–499.

Chapter

11

Reducing Preventable Clinical Deterioration through the Use of a Safety Surveillance Team

Joan S. Roberts and Wendy E. Murchie

Reaching a Tipping Point: 2012

Extending the reach of intensive care unit (ICU) expertise into acute care areas was based on the expanded need for early recognition of clinical deterioration in increasingly more complex medical patients admitted to a regional pediatric hospital.

A brief description of underlying issues will allow a deeper understanding of the development of the structure and function of the safety surveillance team. Seattle Children's Hospital (SCH) is a 278-bed tertiary pediatric medical referral center for Washington and nearby states. Annually, there are more than 75,000 inpatient non-ICU admissions to medical, surgical, cancer, and rehabilitation units. SCH, like other pediatric hospitals, experienced an increase in the acuity of patients over several years along with an increase in technological medical advances and a higher number of chronically ill pediatric patients in the community.

In a retrospective cohort analysis of 28 children's hospitals in the United States, including SCH, there was a 32.5% cumulative increase in hospitalizations of children with a significant chronic condition or complex, progressive disease between 2004 and 2009.[1] In addition, and more specific to our institution, we experienced a significant population growth in our region and an expanding stature of our cardiac, cancer, and craniofacial programs. As a result of these increased demands on the institution, ICU census frequently exceeded bed or staffing capacity, leading to a reverse triage mode of thinking, "healthiest out, sickest in." This allowed higher acuity patients to be discharged to acute care in times of high census, creating a demand for frequent evaluation and readmission to the ICU. ICU staff were often in a crisis mode, with responsibilities both inside and outside of the ICU. Poor communication and documentation of acute care events became the norm. A culture of high ICU "walls" as well as decision-making based on ICU availability and assessment of the need for an ICU level of therapy had solidified. The patient safety and code blue (cardiac arrest) committee reviews suggested that most events had system issues of communication and critical thinking errors.

In response to the increased demand for inpatient ICU beds, SCH built a new building with a planned opening in April 2013, which included a new ICU with 11 additional beds, increasing ICU capacity to 56. This also created a greater demand on the already burdened ICU Rapid Response Team (RRT). The need for increased ICU staffing was apparent, but the wake-up call to change the conceptual model of our ICU response systems took a nudge.

In 2012, there were three unrelated serious adverse events, which drew the focus on patient safety to a new level of importance for administrative leaders. The combination of a call to action to improve patient safety at a time of dynamic facility and staffing changes encouraged leaders to consider a leap in design rather than baby steps.

Defining the Problem

Pulseless arrests in children are rare and associated with very poor outcomes.[2] The mortality rate for pediatric in-hospital and out-of-ICU arrests is reported to be as high as 50%–67%.[3, 4] Due to the low cardiac arrest rates in children, some institutions have chosen to focus on transfers to ICU with critical interventions within a specified time period as predictors of clinical deterioration and end measures for success.[5, 6] These events occur more frequently and can be evaluated to identify earlier opportunities for interventions with clinical relevance for improvement.

After consideration of previously published definitions as metrics, we concluded that none would satisfy our institutional criteria which included inpatient acute care events requiring transfer to ICU that were (1) potentially preventable, (2) clinically relevant, (3) related to mortality and ICU length of stay (LOS), (4) applicable to the entire inpatient non-ICU population, (5) determined by chart review with training but not expert opinion, and (6) frequent enough to measure improvement.

We reviewed the records of acute care inpatients transferred to the ICU over a 15-month timeframe, focusing on the timing and type of interventions, mortality, and LOS. We then developed a clinical metric for deterioration, with exclusion of events that are unlikely to be preventable, such as seizures, and inclusion of events that are likely to be recognized by clinical staff in advance of their occurrence. We called these RESCUE events, which were defined as patients who required transfer to the ICU and resuscitation (noninvasive positive pressure ventilation, mechanical ventilation, or blood pressure support medication) within two hours of ICU admission. The patients identified by this definition had an increased risk for death (13.2% mortality) compared to a 3.4% mortality of ICU admissions from other sources. We reasoned that some of these patients could have been identified and transferred to ICU earlier, which may have allowed mitigation or reversal of the process. By creating a metric related to mortality and associating the work with the concept of preventable harm, we were ready to design interventions to reduce the frequency of these events.

The RISK Program

We performed a comprehensive review of the literature on the efficacy of rapid response systems, focusing on pediatric programs. There were three principal insights that informed our design. First, the work of McCurdy and Wood[7] described the similarity of a rapid response system to the nervous system as composed of two limbs: the afferent limb representing the monitoring, detecting, and activation of the team and the efferent limb representing the actions of the rapid response and code team. This framework enabled the separation of design into two discrete sections: a recognition process and a response process. Second, Duke University Health System reported its implementation of a proactive pediatric ICU "Rover Team" which improved clinical outcomes through earlier interventions, adding a proactive element to identify deterioration early and to intervene efficiently.

The improvement idea conveyed in this work was the a priori identification of high-risk populations automatically generating an evaluation by the response team, rather than waiting for clinical criteria to be met, as well as the clinical outcome metric of readmission to the ICU.[8] Third, Jones et al.[9] analyzed the RRT activation rate and the efficacy of the response team on clinical improvements, finding that organizations with mature RRT systems and a "dose" of 25.8–56.4 calls/1,000 admissions had improved patient outcomes. In other words, RRT events must occur often enough to detect and prevent the untoward events that RRT aims to eliminate. Furthermore, this clarified that RRT activation is not a bad outcome but a means to prevent a bad outcome. The adoption of a definition of a bad outcome was the definition of a RESCUE event as a potential source of preventable harm. These three concepts were invaluable to the design of our program, which we termed **Rec**ognition of **I**llness **S**everity in **K**ids, or RISK.

The components of the RISK program included the proactive surveillance of acute care patients by an ICU expert nurse based on data-driven risk identification, collaboration with acute care teams prior to rapid response activation, rapid response activation process, and ongoing surveillance for patients deemed able to remain in acute care.

Clinical Triggers

Several authors offer strong evidence regarding when to call a RRT; however, few offer valid triggers for instituting a proactive evaluation by a safety surveillance team.[8, 9, 10, 11, 12] Brady et al.[6] created a system to decrease ICU transfers termed as "UNrecognized Situation Awareness Failure Events" (UNSAFE). These events were defined as those requiring transfer to the ICU and resuscitation within 1 hour. A retrospective review of 100 cases meeting the UNSAFE criteria identified five common triggers at their institution. The triggers included: family concerns, high-risk therapies, presence of high early warning scores, watcher or clinician gut feeling, and communication errors. The authors created a thrice daily inpatient safety huddle of healthcare team providers for patients at risk. Patients were proactively identified using these triggers. Through earlier detection, they had a 50% reduction in UNSAFE transfers and serious safety events.

Institutions that identified higher-risk patients demonstrated improvements in readmission rates to the ICU through proactive rounding for up to 48 hours after transfer.[13, 14]

Identifying clinical triggers, or indicators, for proactive huddling and evaluation of a patient by the RISK nurse required familiarity with peer institution experience and reviewing RRT events and ICU transfers from acute care. The most frequent reasons for calling an RRT and for ICU transfer were included as mandatory triggers. These included: nurse, caregiver, or provider concern; unfamiliar care or off clinical pathway patients; patients who had an RRT event within the previous 24 hours; and patients for which an ICU consult occurred in the Emergency Department with subsequent admission to an acute care floor. Several nonmandatory triggers were also identified as possible indications for a safety huddle, including a change in the patient's modified early warning score (Modified Pediatric Early Warning Score [MPEWS]).

Proactive Huddles

We knew proactive huddles were the best method to ensure active surveillance. The hospital had already instituted several huddles into the daily work of the nurses. The proactive RISK huddle needed to address the people, the content, and the timing of the huddles. It was important to observe and learn what routines already existed in the nurses' and providers' daily work. Many hours were spent observing on the acute care units and interacting

RISK Nurse Huddle Process

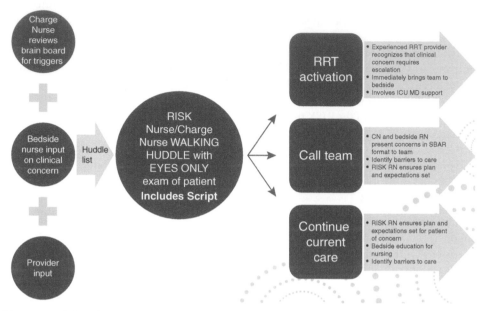

Figure 11.1 RISK RN huddle process
(A black and white version of this figure will appear in some formats. For the color version, refer to the plate section.)

with staff to understand the potential impact of additional huddles. Staff were encouraged to offer potential solutions.

A pilot of one safety huddle per 12-hour shift, with one service, was initiated. This huddle occurred at the start of the day and night shift and included an ICU and acute care charge nurse. This pilot did not result in a reduction of ICU transfers or events but was met with enthusiasm from both charge nurses and staff. A higher degree of camaraderie developed between ICU and acute care staff. There was an additional element of education that occurred for those children with complex illnesses, helping create a positive framework for future work (Figure 11.1).

Designing the Work

Designing the actual work of the RISK nurses and huddle times was the next step to complete. A rapid process design event was held over two days. The 12-person multidisciplinary team comprised providers, a nurse supervisor, and staff nurses from acute care and ICU. The background to the development of the RISK program was presented, along with the data analysis and clinical triggers identified earlier, and the observations and lessons from the pilot huddles.

The team was charged with identifying key participants in the safety huddles, standardization of huddle process and content, creation of a standardized huddle schedule for each acute care unit (Medical, Surgical, Rehabilitation Unit, and Cancer Care Unit), and an audit tool for evaluating the process once it was in place. The design team also collaborated on how the new RISK nurses would evaluate a patient independent of escalation to an RRT.

The team ultimately identified one 12-hour shift huddle per unit and times that worked for each unit's daily schedule. A standard process was created with the charge nurse and bedside nurses first identifying patients using the clinical triggers and placing them on the huddle list, followed by a walking huddle with a RISK nurse. This enhanced RISK nurse visualization of the patient and conversation with the bedside nurse. The design process specified what the RISK nurse's actions during a patient evaluation would entail. Integrating an additional clinical role (the RISK nurse) into an established traditional relationship (bedside nurse, charge nurse, intern/resident/fellow/APP [advanced practice provider, a nurse practitioner or physician assistant], and attending team) was crucial to the success of the program without adding confusion to the decision-making process. The RISK nurse was envisioned to act as a sensory organ of the ICU, to recognize and escalate the need for critical care. This role could easily be misconstrued as interfering with the care plan of the floor team and required deliberate guard rails to prevent antagonism. An important framework was that the RISK nurse be seen in a supportive role, not replacing the work of the bedside or unit charge nurse or supplanting the medical team. The RISK nurse had three options while assessing a patient:

(1) Continue with current care, with patient involvement by RISK nurse limited to assessing the need for critical care consultation. If the patient does not require a higher level of care, the RISK nurse reviews the clinical plan, helps explain the expected trajectory for the patient, and offers education.

(2) Collaborate with the primary team. When the RISK nurse identifies a patient plan or clinical condition as worrisome, then the charge nurse and bedside nurse are coached to present concerns in SBAR (explained further in Chapter 14) format to the primary provider. The RISK nurse will help to identify barriers to care and will ensure the plan and expectations are clear.

(3) Call the RRT. If the patient is requiring urgent care within 10 minutes, an RRT is called and the RISK nurse will assume the RRT ICU nurse role (Figure 11.2).

Building the Team

A job description was designed for this new role, and five full-time equivalent (FTE) nurses from the Critical Care Float Pool were initially interviewed and hired. We chose those from the Critical Care Float Pool as they were ICU nurses with experience in all three ICUs: cardiac, newborn, and pediatric. An essential quality of the RISK nurse was the ability to relate to the acute care nurses' work and to educate others. Most of those hired into the role had either previous acute care experience or experience in a teaching role. Even though thirteen RISK nurses were hired, they each maintained their positions within the Critical Care Float Pool, with 50%–75% of their FTE dedicated to the RISK role. This maintained their ICU experience and added job satisfaction.

Involving the Family Advisory Council was an additional element of the project to ensure insights from caregivers were taken into consideration. In December 2013, key members of the Family Advisory Council were asked to meet on three separate occasions to discuss the design, implementation, and role of the RISK nurse. These parents were integral to presenting the RISK nurse role to families as well as serving on a parent panel for RISK nurse training.

RISK Evaluation Plan

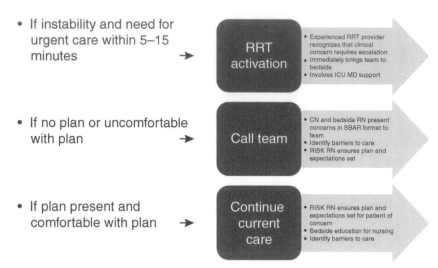

- If instability and need for urgent care within 5–15 minutes → **RRT activation**
  - Experienced RRT provider recognizes that clinical concern requires escalation
  - Immediately brings team to bedside
  - Involves ICU MD support

- If no plan or uncomfortable with plan → **Call team**
  - CN and bedside RN present concerns in SBAR format to team
  - Identify barriers to care
  - RISK RN ensures plan and expectations set

- If plan present and comfortable with plan → **Continue current care**
  - RISK RN ensures plan and expectations set for patient of concern
  - Bedside education for nursing
  - Identify barriers to care

Figure 11.2 RISK RN Evaluation
(A black and white version of this figure will appear in some formats. For the color version, refer to the plate section.)

Training

A 16-hour, two-day didactic and simulation training program was developed for RISK nurses. The didactic classes focused on teamwork, communication, and systematic assessments. A parent panel was included to share ideas and promote open discussion about how to approach caregivers and patients in the acute care units. Simulation of critical events and difficult conversations were added to the training program. Creating a team that effectively communicates and works together is critical to its success.

Key concepts included using SBAR for concise communication between the team members and providers, gaining insight into how others may perceive them and how individual behaviors of each team member can impact others during a stressful clinical situation. We also included simulations that demonstrated clinical and challenging behavior scenarios with team members, providers, patients, and families. The RISK nurses found this training invaluable in preparation for their new role. Implementation of the RISK nurse role occurred in a staggered manner beginning in March 2013. One unit at a time went live to ensure both the nurses and the RISK nurse were effective with "just in time" improvements. Each week an additional unit was added, leading to a full implementation within one month (Figure 11.3).

Documentation

A paper surveillance form was developed for the RISK nurse to document the reason for the huddle or call, the evaluation of the patient, clinical triggers present, and the plan of care. This form included names of those who had been communicated with outside of the RISK nurse and bedside or charge nurse. Included on the form would be the revised plan of care, if indicated, and what signs to watch for indicating clinical deterioration. This form included documentation of education provided to the bedside nurse and the escalation plan.

Day One

Time	Topic
07:00–07:10 hrs	Introductions
07:10–07:45 hrs	Overview of RISK Project • Background • Severe clinical deterioration definition • Daily work overview
07:45–08:45 hrs	Rapid Response • MPEWS Tool • Escalation Algorithm & RISK RN • Role and Responsibilities • Event Record
08:45–09:00 hrs	**Break**
09:00–10:00 hrs	Teamwork and Communication • Learn and understand how to use a structured communication technique to facilitate effective communication
10:00–11:00 hrs	Systematic Approach Algorithm • Why it is important • Systematic Approach Algorithm • Simulation/Practice
11:00–11:45 hrs	**Lunch**
11:45–13:00 hrs	Parent Prespective
13:00–14:00 hrs	RISK Huddles • Roles & Responsibilities • Surveillance Tool
14:00–14:15 hrs	**Break**
14:15–15:00 hrs	MPEWS Escalation Algorithm Pilot • Objectives • Algorithm review • Actions • Audit
15:00 hrs	Wrap up

Day Two

Time	Topic
07:00–11:00 hrs	Simulation Scenarios
11:00–12:00 hrs	Break for Lunch
12:00–15:00 hrs	IV Training

Figure 11.3 RISK RN Training
(A black and white version of this figure will appear in some formats. For the color version, refer to the plate section.)

House-wide education about the new RISK program, triggers, and huddles was provided to both acute care nurses and providers in January and February 2013. In September 2013, after several months of design work and five months following the RISK nurse implementation, this form became a part of the electronic medical record, making it readily accessible to nurses and providers (Figure 11.4).

RISK RN Surveillance

Reason for RISK RN Evaluation
- ☑ RN/Provider/Parent concern
- ☐ RRT in last 24 hours
- ☐ Unfamiliar or off-pathway care
- ☐ MPEWS > = 5 in first 24 hours
- ☐ ED-ICU consult
- ☐ Other:

RISK RN Evaluation
Called to bedside for self limiting tachyarrythmias lasting only 30 seconds × 2. Patient sleeping and without complaint. Other vital signs and perfusion within normal range.

RISK RN Recommendation
- ○ Continue with current plan
- ● Notify team to clarify or modify plan (specify)
- ○ Call RRT & notify team to clarify/modify plan

Summary of Team Discussion
Team called to bedside to confirm ECG strip arrhythmias. 12 lead ECG performed. Team advised bedside RN to give lasix as ordered in the morning and will consider ordering lytes for am labs.

Communication Plan
- ☑ Primary contact MD/NP   ☑ RN
- ☑ Secondary contact MD/NP   ☑ Acute Care Charge nurse
- ☑ Attending
- ☑ Family
- ☑ ICU Charge nurse
- ☐ Respiratory Therapist

Recommended Update to Nursing Care Plan
Increases VS to q2h × 8hrs overnight. Include perfusion checks with VS and document in IView. Print ECG strips every shift and place in chart. If arrythmias occur, print strip and perform VS and perfusion check

Signs of deterioration to watch for
If hemodynamically unstable (low BP, CR >3sec, cool extremities, possibly altered LOC) call Code Blue. If tachyarrythmias occur again and hemodynamically stable (normal BP, CR <3sec, warm extremities) call cardiac transplant fellow and RRT.

RISK RN Actions
- ☑ Education
- ☐ IV start
- ☐ Suction patient
- ☐ Transport to Radiology
- ☐ Other:

Education Provided
- ☐ NP suction
- ☐ Fever management
- ☐ Airway positioning
- ☑ Signs/symptoms shock
- ☐ Signs/symptoms respiratory distress/failure
- ☐ Signs/symptoms increased ICP
- ☐ Other

Is Follow Up Needed?
- ○ No follow up needed
- ● Next follow up due

Next Follow Up Due   11/18/2013 ◌ ⌄   0600 ◌

Figure 11.4 RISK RN surveillance form
(A black and white version of this figure will appear in some formats. For the color version, refer to the plate section.)

Additional Design Work

In addition to the RISK nurse role, we continued to do further data analysis on our MPEWS following the start of the RISK program. This showed a correlation between an increased risk of RESCUE event and an MPEWS of five or greater in the first 24 hours of admission or transfer to acute care, as well as an increasing MPEWS score, calculated based on the patient's previous scores, after the first 24 hours of admission. An automatic trigger was built to alert the RISK nurse and the patient's primary provider by a text page. A mandatory RISK nurse evaluation within two hours of the alert, an increase in the frequency of vital signs and focused assessments for 8 hours by the bedside nurse, and a notification to the patient's primary provider were implemented and added to the RISK nurse work.

An electronic dashboard was created for the RISK nurse workflow in the electronic medical record. We worked on this in the months following the RISK nurse implementation.

The dashboard had three categories of patients being watched by the RISK nurse: those who have had an RRT or Code and stayed on the floor, those with two MPEWS trigger alerts, and those identified in a huddle or through nurse or provider concern. This dashboard set a time for follow-up and displayed this time for nurses and providers. Real-time MPEWS are displayed and automatically updated every three minutes to show real-time acuity of those being watched by the RISK nurse. This dashboard allows anyone to access

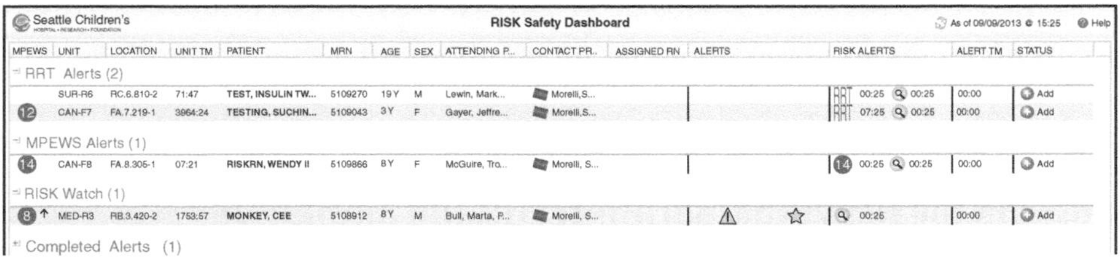

Figure 11.5 RISK RN dashboard
All images created by the chapter authors, no permission required from Seattle Children's Hospital
(A black and white version of this figure will appear in some formats. For the color version, refer to the plate section.)

trending MPEWS scores, surveillance documentation, and patient charts of any patient followed by the RISK nurse (Figure 11.5).

Outcome Measurements

The pre-RISK and post-RISK periods of time were compared, with each timespan containing a full year to ensure inclusion of the normal variance of RESCUE events during the year (such as respiratory season), with exclusion of the three-month gap during implementation of the RISK nurse to allow integration of the role.

What happened to the number of rapid response activations, ICU transfers, and RESCUE events?

Rapid response activations increased from 10.3 activations/1,000 to 12.6/1,000 acute care inpatient days, an increase of 18%. The actual number of RRT calls increased by 44.8%. The number and rate of patients transferring to the ICU also increased from 4.9 to 7.2 transfers/1,000 acute care inpatient days. There was an estimated 35% of this increased transfer rate associated with protocol changes outside the RISK program. The percentage of rapid response activations that resulted in transfer to the ICU was unchanged (57% in both groups). The number and rate of RESCUE events fell from 98 to 60 actual events, a 39% decrease, and the RESCUE event rate decreased from 1.7 per 1,000 to 1.1 per 1,000 acute care inpatient days.

What was the work of the RISK nurse?

Five FTE nurse salaries were devoted to the project with training of 13 nurses for the RISK nurse role. The electronic safety surveillance form and dashboard allowed us to evaluate the work the RISK nurse performed. The RISK nurse performed an average of 15 patient evaluations in a 12-hour shift in addition to approximately one RRT event per 12-hour shift. In addition to this work, the RISK nurse educated the bedside nurse on signs of clinical deterioration. Evaluation and care of the patient with respiratory distress were the clinical subjects with the largest amount of allotted time taught by the RISK nurses. The busiest time of day was between 3 and 7 p.m. The majority of MPEWS alerts occurred during this time, which correlates to the influx of PACU and ED patients admitted to acute care. RISK nurse watch evaluations were highest between 11 p.m. and 3 a.m. Many new nurses are on the night shift, and this increase in RISK nurse evaluations may be a result of this inexperience. Overall, there was no difference in the workload during day or night shifts. Weekdays were busier than weekends.

How did the RISK program affect LOS and mortality?

The mortality rate fell for all patients transferring, as would be expected with a higher rate of transfer and a more conservative approach to early transfer. For patients with a RESCUE event, the pre-RISK mortality of 14.3% fell to 12.5% post-RISK implementation. For non-RESCUE event patients (those who required transfer to the ICU but did not require resuscitation), the mortality rate also dropped from 6.9% to 6.0%. Similarly, the LOS for both RESCUE event and non-RESCUE event transfers decreased from 11 to 10 days (9%) and 7 to 6 days (14%). These results suggest that our practice changed overall rather than in an isolated manner and that our approach shifted to more frequent, somewhat shorter ICU stays with the ability to intervene earlier in critical illness.

How well were patients identified who deteriorated?

In the post-RISK time period, we were able to assess the activation of 772 RRT events. Nurse concern was the primary trigger of activation most often (58% of the time), with automatic triggers and provider triggers much less frequent (13% of the time). RRTs activated by nursing had a much higher likelihood of a RESCUE event (20%) than those activated by a provider (10%). One implication drawn from this may be that when nursing and providers agree, escalation is more rapid and efficient.

The RISK nurse was involved up to 8 hours prior to activation in 24% of RRT calls. Of these RRTs, 27 (42.2%) were RESCUE events. The 28-day mortality rate in those with RISK nurse involvement was higher at 14.8% than those where the RISK nurse was not involved at 5.4%. This may be because the RISK nurse was involved with the higher acuity patients earlier. The RISK nurse was asked to evaluate patients outside of an RRT most frequently by the automated MPEWS 5 or greater alert 51% of the time. The other RISK nurse evaluations occurred 34.7% of the time for nurse, caregiver, or provider concern, and only 7.8% for a previous RRT event within the last 24 hours. Overall, the mandatory clinical triggers initiated 80% of the RRT calls and RISK nurse evaluations. Taken together, our experience suggests that automatic triggers are correctly identifying the patients (the efferent limb), but that our RISK nurse and RRT process have not been as effective in appropriately transferring the correct patients (the afferent limb).

How was the program received by staff?

Six months following the initiation of the RISK nurse, all acute care nurses were surveyed. The goals of the survey were to understand the following from the nurses who were working with the RISK nurses:

Overall satisfaction with RISK nurse

Percentage of correct understanding as to when to call the RISK nurse versus RRT

Percentage of inclusion of primary team awareness when requesting RISK nurse

Perception of improved patient care

Perception of gained education

Perception of improved safety

The outcomes of the survey were exciting. There was 100% overall satisfaction with the RISK program and a perception of improved patient care and safety. The survey provided insight into education opportunities to include the primary provider when the RISK nurse was being utilized for a patient, as well as reminders on when to include a patient in a RISK huddle. Data demonstrated improvement in patient care and a reduction in barriers to calling for help.

How does this program affect cost?

The budget for this project included the RISK nurses' and project leaders' time as well as the telecommunications, data analytics services or IT, and education required to implement the project. The education and communication budgets were required for approximately two months preimplementation, whereas the RISK nurses, project leads, and data analytics/IT budget were required throughout the project until the program was fully operationalized. The information technology aspect of the budget was incremental and only required for startup of the electronic medical record dashboard and surveillance forms.

Analysis of LOS and cost information from patients requiring transfer to the ICU was performed. Thirty patients in both comparison groups (pre-RISK and post-RISK) were randomly chosen, 15 from each event group (transfer to ICU with RESCUE event and transfer to ICU without RESCUE event). Actual financial costs of this total cohort of 60 patients were obtained, and all costs adjusted to reflect 2010 values. The cost per day of a non-RESCUE event patient was $3,523, whereas the cost per day of a RESCUE event patient was $5,175. All ICU transfers were also evaluated as to whether they were protocol-driven transfers. The RISK program would not have influenced protocol-driven transfers since these transfers occur due to hospital protocol and were accounted for in the estimation model.

The cost of ICU transfers, including both non-RESCUE event and RESCUE event transfers, in 2012 pre-RISK implementation was $10,104,000. We performed a cost projection, which assumed the RISK program had not been implemented, and applied the baseline rates of transfer and LOS to the cohort of patients in the post-RISK 12-month period. The projected cost without the RISK program was $10,104,000. Next, we compared the actual costs of the post-RISK cohort, which included more patients admitted to the hospital and more patients transferred to the ICU, but fewer RESCUE events and shorter LOS. Our analysis concluded that for the first year, the RISK program cost the hospital $2,792,000 and saved $3,509,000, with a net saving of $717,000. This cost analysis fails to include the potential savings inherent in the mitigation or prevention of life-threatening events. For 100 RESCUE events, 15 patients will not survive to discharge, so potentially reducing these events provides a huge saving in human years.

Summary

With establishment of a pediatric safety surveillance program, there were substantial reductions in the number of RESCUE events and mortality rates. In addition, increased safety surveillance was associated with an increase in staff satisfaction and ICU-acute care collaboration. The cost of this program was warranted by the reduction in preventable harm and immeasurable lives saved.

References

1. Berry J, Hall M, Hall D, Kuo D, Cohen E, Agrawal R, and Neff J. Inpatient growth and resource use in 28 children's hospitals: A longitudinal, multi-institutional study. *Journal of the American Medical Association Pediatrics.* 2013;167:e559–e565.

2. Nadkarni V, Larkin G, Peberdy M, Carey S, Kaye W, Mancini M, and Berg R. First documented rhythm and clinical outcome from in-hospital cardiac arrest among children and adults. *Journal of American Medical Association.* 2006;295:50–57.

3. Reis A, Nadkarni V, Perondi M, Grisi S, and Berg R. A prospective investigation into the epidemiology of in-hospital pediatric cardiopulmonary resuscitation using the international Utstein reporting style. *Pediatrics.* 2002;109:200–209.

4. Suominen P, Olkkola K, Voipio V, Korpela R, Palo R, and Rasanen J. Utstein style reporting of in-hospital paediatric cardiopulmonary resuscitation. *Resuscitation.* 2000;45:17–25.

5. Bonafide C, Roberts K, Priestly M, Tibbetts K, Huang E, and Keren R. Development of a pragmatic measure for evaluating and optimizing rapid response systems. *Pediatrics.* 2012;129:1–8.

6. Brady P, Muething S, Kotagal U, Ashby M, Gallagher R, Hall D, and Wheeler D. Improving situation awareness to reduce unrecognized clinical deterioration and serious safety events. *Pediatrics.* 2012;131:e298–e308.

7. McCurdy T and Wood S. Rapid response systems: Identification and management of the "prearrest state." *Emergency Medical Clinics in North America.* 2012;30:141–152.

8. Hueckel R, Turi J, Cheifetz I, Mericle J, Meliones J, and Mistry K. Beyond rapid response teams: Instituting a "rover team" improves the management of at-risk patients, facilitates proactive interventions, and improves outcomes. *Advances in Patient Safety: New Directions and Alternative Approaches.* Henriksen K, Battles J, Keyes M, et al., eds., Rockville, MD, Agency for Healthcare Research and Quality (US), 2008. www.ncbi.nlm.nih.gov/books/nbk43680/

9. Jones D, Dunbar N, and Bellomo R. Clinical deterioration in hospital inpatients: The need for another paradigm shift. *Medical Journal of Australia.* 2012;196:97–100.

10. Daly M, Powers J, Orto V, Rogers M, Dickinson T, Fabris M, and Honan M. Innovative solutions: Leading the way. *Dimensions of Critical Care Nursing.* 2007;126:15–20.

11. DeVita M. Medical emergency teams: Deciphering clues to crises in hospitals. *Critical Care.* 2005;9:325–326.

12. Jansen J and Cuthbertson B. Detecting critical illness outside the ICU: The role of track and trigger systems. *Current Opinion in Critical Care.* 2010;16:1–7.

13. Butcher B, Vittinghoff E, Maselli J, and Auerbach A. Impact of proactive rounding by a rapid response team on patient outcomes at an academic medical center. *Journal of Hospital Medicine.* 2013;8:7–12.

14. Caffin C, Linton S, and Pellegrini J. Introduction of a liaison nurse role in a tertiary paediatric ICU. *Intensive and Critical Care Nursing.* 2007;23:226–233.

Chapter

12 Nursing Perspective in Patient Safety: Quality, Safety, and Advocacy

Cindy B. Katz

Introduction

Nursing presence at the bedside has long been associated with patient care, positive outcomes, and patient advocacy. The nurse is the primary caregiver in the hospital setting while also maintaining roles of patient advocate, teacher, supportive listener, and protector of the patient's physical and mental well-being. The patient needs to be able to trust the intentions of the nurse, perhaps more than any other healthcare professional.[1] The presence of a nurse, a key member of the healthcare team, has demonstrated improved outcomes whether providing care in an outpatient setting or at the bedside in a hospital.

Nurses have long been considered the most trustworthy of all professionals surveyed annually in the US, leading the rankings for the past 19 years.[2] Nurses' honesty and ethical standards were recognized as high or very high by those surveyed without significant differences in respondent age, race, or gender.

Nurses are actively involved at the patient bedside during life's most challenging and vulnerable moments. The act of being present allows the patient to perceive a meaningful exchange between the patient and the nurse[1] and demonstrates the science and the art of expert nursing care.

The earned trust of nurses by patients is built on a foundation of science and education. Modern-day nursing care is based on the evolution of evidence-based practice (EBP). Evidence-based practice origins are found in the earliest efforts in the 1850's by Florence Nightingale, considered the founder of nursing. Her insistence on improving hygiene practice at the bedside and in the hospital caring for soldiers during the Crimean War reduced the hospital death rate by two-thirds.[3, 4] Using data and science, Nightingale collected clean towels and clothing, eating utensils and soap and led the nurses in cleaning up the kitchen and hospital wards. She understood the principles of statistics and demonstrated that actions led to improved outcomes.[5]

Patient Safety and Advocacy

In the historic Institute of Medicine's report "To Err is Human," the role of safety systems and human factors were addressed in Chapter 8, setting performance standards and expectations for patient safety. Included in this noteworthy book were recommendations for creating nonpunitive environments and systems for reporting errors and accidents and managing work in teams similar to aviation. Encouragement to speak up connected patient safety and advocacy with the expectations that institutions must support their workers in identifying and addressing error without fear of formal or informal reprisal.[6]

Attention to patient advocacy and speaking up has gained attention in healthcare with the awareness of lessons learned and improved outcomes in the aviation industry. Aviation addressed the volume of unexpected incidents, crashes, and near misses involving human error through the development of Crew or Cockpit Resource Management (CRM).[7]

In the 1970's, more than 70% of air crashes involved human error rather than weather or equipment failure. Listening to black box recordings recovered from crash-sites demonstrated someone knew something but did not clearly communicate due to a presumed deference to authority and reluctance to speak up. Over time, CRM has evolved and is now a standard part of flight training by the aviation industry, including flight crew, pilots, and ground staff.[8, 9] CRM training includes situational awareness, communication skills, teamwork, task allocation and decision-making.

Silence or reluctance to speak up when someone on the team knew something, resulted in poor outcomes. In healthcare, root cause analyses (See Chapter 6) have demonstrated inadequate communication to be the most frequent root cause of errors.[10] Not speaking up can lead to patient harm.

Speaking Up

Much has been written about the role of nurses in patient safety, and in particular, the role of a nurse as a patient advocate. Speaking up is associated with characteristics of advocacy, vigilance, protection, and representing those who cannot speak. Nurses benefit from learning and practicing CRM skills, including speaking up, through coached and practiced simulation (Chapter 2). Through discussion and presentation of real-life scenarios, and interventions focused on increasing speaking up behaviors, nurses demonstrated and enhanced their ability to speak up for patient safety.[11]

Utilizing communication tools such as SBAR and Read-Backs (See Chapter 14), known as error prevention tools, have contributed to a reduction in errors, improved teamwork, and improved patient outcomes. Using communication and simulation tools has given nurses and team members caring for patients the training and practice to speak up and advocate for patient safety.

Organizational culture is a strong predictor of speaking up. Speaking up affirms nurses' moral courage and is influenced by personal, generational and organizational culture.[12, 14] The evolution of evidence-based practice has demonstrated the connection between nursing leadership, patient safety, adverse events, and the presence and advocacy of the nurse. Patient outcomes, such as mortality, length of stay, falls, catheter use, and pain management are related to nursing leadership. Positive leadership behaviors may be associated with quality care or more effective teamwork.[15]

Evidence based practice of nursing has accelerated since the time of Nightingale and plays a critical role in nursing practice. Whether measuring outcomes in health, safety, or quality, the nurse will continue to be a strong influencer.[4]

References

1. Zyblock DM. Nursing presence in contemporary nursing practice. *Nursing Forum*. April–June 2010;45(2):120–24.

2. Gaines K. Nurses Ranked Most Trusted Profession 19 Years in a Row. Nurse. Org: January 19, 2021. https://nurse.org/ articles/nursing-ranked-most-honest-profession/ (Accessed 29/05/2021).

3. Editors, History.com. Florence Nightingale. April 17, 2020. www.history .com/topics/womens-history/florence-nightingale-1 (Accessed 29/05/2021).

4. McMenamin A, Sun C, and Prufeta P, et al. The evolution of evidence-based practice. *Nursing Management*. September 2019;50(9):14–19.

5. Fee E and Garofalo M. Florence Nightingale and the Crimean War. *American Journal of Public Health*. August 2011;100(9):1591.

6. Kohn LT, Corrigan JM, Donaldson MS, eds., To Err Is Human. Institute of Medicine (US) Committee on Quality of Health Care in America. Washington, DC, National Academies Press; 2000. www.ncbi.nlm.nih.gov/books/NBK225174/ (Accessed 1/11/2020).

7. AeroGuard. What Is Crew Resource Management (CRM)? August 10, 2020. www.flyaeroguard.com/blog/what-is-crew-resource-management/ (Accessed 30/05/2021).

8. American Psychological Association, Science in Action. Safer Air Travel Through Crew Resource Management. February 2014. www.apa.org/action/resources/research-in-action/crew (Accessed 20/05/2021).

9. U.S. Departments of Transportation Federal Aviation Administration Advisory Circular: Crew Resource Management Training, AC 120-51E. January 22, 2004. www.faa.gov/documentlibrary/media/advisory_circular/ac120-51e.pdf (Accessed 31/07/2021).

10. The Joint Commission's Annual report on Quality and Safety 2007. www.jointcommission.org/-/media/tjc/documents/accred-and-cert/hap/annual-report/2007_annual_reportpdf.pdf?db=web&hash=2092D322E8296BCE340B5FF331BDAD82 (Accessed 30/05/2021).

11. Sayre MM, McNeese-Smith D, Phillips LR, et al. A strategy to improve nurses speaking up and collaborating for patient safety. *JONA: The Journal of Nursing Administration*. 2012;42(10):458–460.

12. Rainer, J. Speaking up: Factors and issues in nurses advocating for patients when patients are in jeopardy. *Journal of Nursing Care Quality*. 2015;30(1):53–62.

13. Nsiah C, Siakwa M, and Ninnoni J. Registered Nurses' description of patient advocacy in the clinical setting. *Nursing Open*. 2019;6(3):1124–1132. https://doi.org/10.1002/nop2.307 (Accessed 7/19/22).

14. Rainer JB, and Schneider JK. Testing a model of speaking up in nursing. *JONA: The Journal of Nursing Administration*. June 2020;50(6):349–354.

15. Wong CA, Cumming GG, and Ducharme L. The relationship between nursing leadership and patient outcomes: A systematic review update. *Journal of Nursing Management*. 2013;21:709–724.

Checklists and Transitions of Care: A How-To Guide

Daniel K. W. Low

Six Sigma, a commonly applied framework within high-reliability operations, strives to reduce defect rates to under 3.4 per million events. This is achievable in healthcare if we leverage what human factors teach us with the right process engineering, deployed in a culture which supports these tools and concepts.

Checklists

Checklists are simple tools with proven efficacy in many high-risk industries such as aviation.

There are two main types of checklists: read-do checklists and challenge-response checklists. The concepts underpinning them are fundamental to understanding how to create and use them. Barriers to the successful implementation of checklists are discussed further in Chapter 15, along with some suggestions as to how to overcome these difficulties.

Read-Do Checklists

As the name suggests, "read" an item from the checklist and "do" the action associated with it.

A common example of this type is the anesthesia machine checklist. The first item from the ASA anesthesia machine check is "Verify Auxiliary Oxygen Cylinder and Self-inflating Manual Ventilation Device are Available & Functioning." The accompanying action would be to verify the oxygen cylinder is attached, check its pressure, and verify a self-inflating bag valve mask device is available and functional.

Challenge-Response Checklists

These are typically performed by two people: one issues the challenge and the other is responsible for verifying that a task *has been* performed. The "patient flow checklist" extensively used at the Bellevue Surgery Center at Seattle Children's Hospital is an example of a challenge-response checklist. The patient's surgical journey starts in the induction room, transitions into the operating room, and then moves into the postanesthesia care unit. Each move has been identified as a risk point (Figure 13.1). Checklists were developed for each stage of that journey to ensure (a) before a move, the patient and equipment are configured correctly for transport and (b) immediately following a move, the patient and the equipment are configured correctly.

An example of one of the checklists is the operating room arrival. As the patient is moved into the operating room, the team will turn on oxygen flow, set the vaporizer, con-

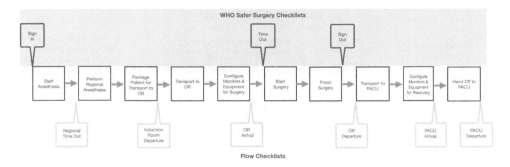

Figure 13.1 Patient Flow Checklist schematic indicating times when checklists are used
(A black and white version of this figure will appear in some formats. For the color version, refer to the plate section.)

nect the monitors, move the airway supplies and medications from the stretcher to the anesthesia machine, and secure the operating room (lock the doors from the induction room). These actions might seem so obvious and automatic that one might question the need for a checklist.

Human factors teach us that as tasks become "routine," they are performed almost unconsciously yet unreliably. Think about when you wake up in the morning on a typical work day. You might brush your teeth, have breakfast, grab your ID badge, wallet, keys, and phone; and head out the door, locking it on the way out. Most readers have forgotten one or more of those actions this year, which approximates to a 1:300 failure rate. A 2013 study by Post-it found the average adult forgets four things a day of that gravity.[1]

Conceptually, the patient flow checklists are no different from checklists developed in aviation for different phases of normal flight: preflight, push back/engine start, after engine start, taxi, before takeoff, after takeoff, climb, descent, and approach. For flight safety, it would be unacceptable to have the crew perform critical tasks from memory; hence, checklists are now required and culturally expected.

Most anesthesiologists know of a case where "pre-oxygenation" occurred with air, "antibiotics" were given that were just saline, or oxygen was not turned on immediately after arrival in the operating room. All "routine" tasks, yet certainly not performed at Six Sigma (3.4 per million) defect rates.

So How Do We Improve Our Defect Rates?

Democratize the knowledge

The regional time-out checklist (Figure 13.2) can be used as an example of this. The last line item is "maximum dose?" It is asked by a nurse to the anesthesiologist who must respond with a volume of local anesthetic (ropivacaine) they are about to draw up. The physician makes a mental weight-based calculation and then converts that drug mass into a volume. The nurse uses a cognitive aid to read off the maximum permitted volume for that particular local anesthetic and that patient's weight and verifies that the maximum dose is not breached. Before deploying the cognitive aid, the team

Regional Block Time-Out
Seattle Children's Main Operating Room

1. Anesthesiologist starts time-out
2. Starred (*) response first
3. RN initiates all other challenges
4. Emphasize all participants must verbally agree
5. If regional time-out is done simultaneously with surgical time-out, start with "block type" after surgical time-out is complete

6. Block site MUST be marked by the person performing the block. This can occur at any time, including during the time-out. Emphasize that the person marking should verify the location with a primary source such as constent. Bilateral and midline blocks do not need to be marked.

7. New local anesthetic dosing table

Challenge	Regional Response	OR Anesthesia Response	RN Response
Identify	Matches Consent	Matches CIS	Reads Wrist Band
Consent	Reads Consent		
Surgical Site	Marked and Matches Consent	"Agree"	"Agree"
*** START HERE IF COMBINING WITH SURGICAL TIME OUT ***			
Block Type	States Block Type(s)		
Block Site	Marks or Verifies Mark At Block Sites(s)	"Correct"	"Correct"
Allergies		Y/N and Specify	
Skin Prep Restrictions		Y/N and Specify	
Anticoagulation		Y/N and Specify	
Medication	State Medication Concentration (%), and Total Planned Dose (mL)	State Patient Weight	Verify Max Dose from Table / View Drug Vial; Verify % and Expiration Date
	Draw up medication		
Any Concerns?	STATE CONCERN		

Figures 13.2 Regional Timeout Checklist
(A black and white version of this figure will appear in some formats. For the color version, refer to the plate section.)

conducted a survey of the perioperative nurses. Almost none of them were confident they could calculate a toxic dose of either 0.2% or 0.5% ropivacaine for a pediatric patient. Consequently, almost none of them felt they were able to raise a concern that a dose was too much. After deploying this simple reference table (Figure 13.3) to determine ceiling doses, the same survey was issued; 100% of nurses felt confident in calling a ceiling dose and 100% felt able to challenge an anesthesiologist if they were about to exceed that dose.

Function as a team, not as a collection of individuals

The introduction of a simple reference table closed the knowledge gap for a specific task: administration of local anesthetic in the context of regional anesthesia. Safe administration of regional anesthesia at Bellevue Surgery Center is now a team activity with team responsibility to ensure the correct block is being performed, on the correct limb, which has been correctly marked in accordance with the consent form.

Reduce hierarchy in the team

Continuing with the above example, it would not work if the culture did not support this workflow. If a nurse is not able to call out an error (perceived or real), then the team will eventually fail. There are a few practical ways to help flatten the hierarchy: (a) first names for everyone (b) have the nurse run the checklists – the nurse issues the "challenge" in the challenge-response-style checklists. That puts them in the situational leadership role which helps create the "one-team, many voices" concept. Finally, putting the knowledge out there publicly for all to see (on a poster, for example) closes knowledge gaps which in turn closes "power gaps" between team members.

Maximum Dose Ropivacaine Plain OR Bupivacaine with Epinephrine 0.2% - 0.5% (3 mg/kg)			
Weight (kg)	**0.2% (ml)**	**0.25% (mL)**	**0.5% (mL)**
3	4	3	1
4	6	4	`2
5	7	6	3
6	9	7	3
7	10	8	4
8	12	9	4
9	13	10	5
10	15	12	6
12	18	14	7
14	21	16	8
16	24	19	9
18	27	21	10
20	30	24	12
22	33	26	13
24	36	28	14
26	39	31	15
28	42	33	16
30	45	36	18
32	48	38	19
34	51	40	20
36	54	43	21
38	57	45	22
40	60	48	24
42	63	50	25
44	66	52	26
46	69	55	27
48	72	57	28
50	75	60	30
52	78	62	31
54	81	64	32
56	84	67	33
58	87	69	34
60	90	72	36
>60	1.5 mL/kg	1.2 mL/kg	0.6 mL/kg
Note: Maximum Dose for Bupivacaine Plain is 2.5 mg/kg: 1 mL/kg (0.25%) or 0.5 mL/kg (0.5%)			

Figure 13.3 Regional Anesthesia Reference Dosing Table
(A black and white version of this figure will appear in some formats. For the color version, refer to the plate section.)

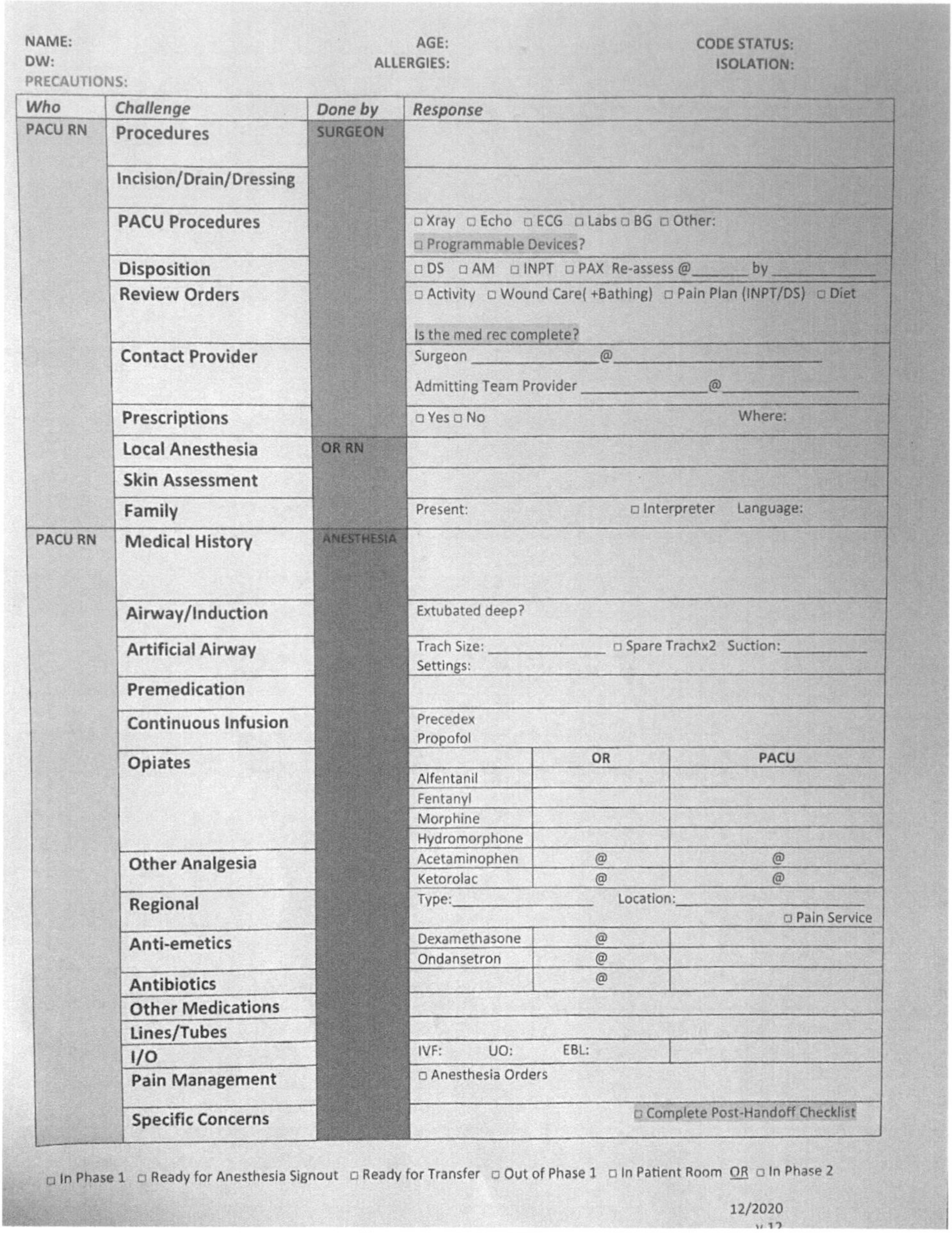

NAME: AGE: CODE STATUS:
DW: ALLERGIES: ISOLATION:
PRECAUTIONS:

Who	Challenge	Done by	Response
PACU RN	Procedures	SURGEON	
	Incision/Drain/Dressing		
	PACU Procedures		□ Xray □ Echo □ ECG □ Labs □ BG □ Other: □ Programmable Devices?
	Disposition		□ DS □ AM □ INPT □ PAX Re-assess @_____ by _____
	Review Orders		□ Activity □ Wound Care(+Bathing) □ Pain Plan (INPT/DS) □ Diet Is the med rec complete?
	Contact Provider		Surgeon _____@_____ Admitting Team Provider _____@_____
	Prescriptions		□ Yes □ No Where:
	Local Anesthesia	OR RN	
	Skin Assessment		
	Family		Present: □ Interpreter Language:
PACU RN	Medical History	ANESTHESIA	
	Airway/Induction		Extubated deep?
	Artificial Airway		Trach Size: _____ □ Spare Trachx2 Suction:_____ Settings:
	Premedication		
	Continuous Infusion		Precedex Propofol

			OR	PACU
	Opiates	Alfentanil		
		Fentanyl		
		Morphine		
		Hydromorphone		
	Other Analgesia	Acetaminophen	@	@
		Ketorolac	@	@
	Regional	Type:_____ Location:_____		□ Pain Service
	Anti-emetics	Dexamethasone	@	
		Ondansetron	@	
	Antibiotics		@	
	Other Medications			
	Lines/Tubes			
	I/O	IVF: UO: EBL:		
	Pain Management	□ Anesthesia Orders		
	Specific Concerns		□ Complete Post-Handoff Checklist	

□ In Phase 1   □ Ready for Anesthesia Signout   □ Ready for Transfer   □ Out of Phase 1   □ In Patient Room OR □ In Phase 2

12/2020
v. 12

Figure 13.4 PACU Handoff Checklist
(A black and white version of this figure will appear in some formats. For the color version, refer to the plate section.)

Reducing Errors by Using Cross-checks

Staying with the example of avoiding local anesthetic toxicity by using a team and check-list approach, we will assume that the error rate for a single physician performing mental arithmetic is 1:1,000 (which is about 10 years of a career, if 100 blocks are performed a year). The error rate for reading off the reference chart should be less, since it is just read-

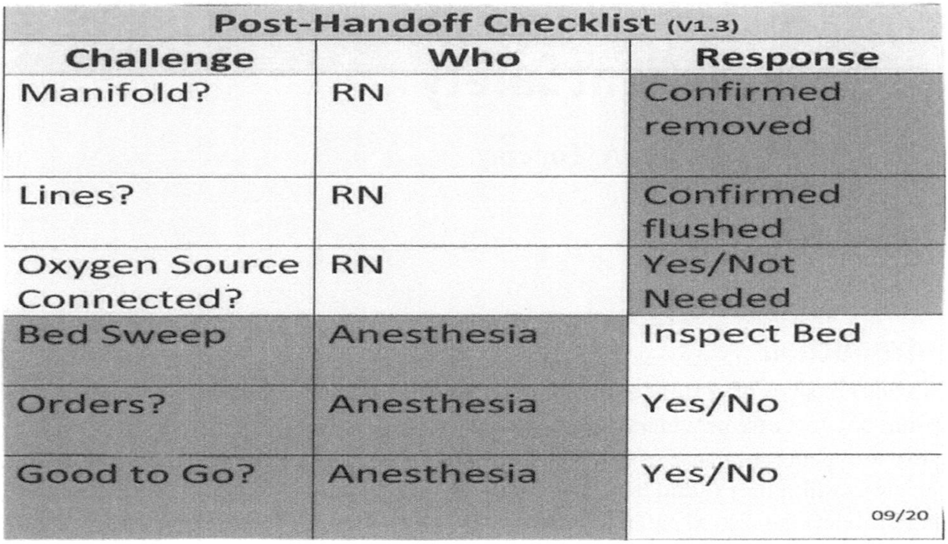

Post-Handoff Checklist (v1.3)		
Challenge	**Who**	**Response**
Manifold?	RN	Confirmed removed
Lines?	RN	Confirmed flushed
Oxygen Source Connected?	RN	Yes/Not Needed
Bed Sweep	Anesthesia	Inspect Bed
Orders?	Anesthesia	Yes/No
Good to Go?	Anesthesia	Yes/No

09/20

Figure 13.5 PACU Departure Checklist
(A black and white version of this figure will appear in some formats. For the color version, refer to the plate section.)

ing a volume, cross-referenced with a weight. Let us assume 1:10,000 for that error. The theoretical combined error rate that will reach a patient would be $1:1,000 \times 1:10,000 = 1:10,000,000$. That is the effect of a true independent cross-check.

Transitions of Care

Patient handoffs are widely accepted as being high-risk points for information being miscommunicated, misunderstood, or not passed on. The best handoff of care occurs at the patient bedside, face-to-face between the person handing off care and the person taking over care. At Seattle Children's Hospital, the standard process is to have a representative of the surgical team, anesthesia team, and operative nursing team accompany the patient from the operating room to the postanesthesia care unit (PACU). The handoff occurs after the patient is monitored and the team agrees it is safe to start. The order in which the teams communicate with the PACU RN is predetermined; the elements required from each team are also predetermined. The handoff checklist is shown in Figure 13.4. When designing the handoff checklist, the teams worked hard to ensure the noise-to-signal ratio was as low as possible.

After recovery, if the patient is being admitted, the surgical RN comes to the PACU to receive a direct face-to-face handoff of care with an opportunity to verify the information being given and to ask clarifying questions. This handoff occurs before the patient is transported to the surgical floor.

In addition, just prior to leaving the bedside in PACU, the RN leads a final checklist to make sure that the patient is safe, the RN has all of the orders and information that they need and that no medications or equipment have inadvertently been left in the patient's bed (Figure 13.5).

Reference

1. Conner J. The average person forgets 4 things a day; 2013. Available at: https:// us105fm.com/the-average-person-forgets-4-things-a-day/ (Accessed 7/4/22).

Communication Tools to Improve Patient Safety

Kristina A. Toncray

Introduction

In a 2007 analysis of sentinel events, the Joint Commission noted "inadequate communication between care providers or between care providers and patients/families is consistently the main root cause of sentinel events."[1] In addition, Vermeir et al. conducted a review in which they found that poor communication can lead to not only compromised patient safety but also to patient dissatisfaction and economic losses via provider rework and investigations of issues.[2]

We communicate and with one another constantly in healthcare: with other physicians and with nursing staff, and to our patients. Proper communication is an absolute necessity in order to provide high-quality care. High-functioning teams in healthcare and elsewhere use tools that help clarify their thoughts and increase the quality of their communication. Handoffs, presented in Chapter 13, help us in clarifying our communication. This chapter presents other tools that can aid in improving our communication and making our messages to one another clear.

Communication is influenced by a number of factors. Personality, training, hierarchy, and culture all play a role. How one's communication efforts were received by others in the past, for example, affects one's current and future communication styles. Someone who has been treated poorly in the past for sharing a concern is less likely to speak up in the future. Setting expectations about standard communication tools within a system, then, can help improve team dynamics and patient care.

Most physicians did not take courses in medical school that addressed the proper way to communicate to ensure that they are understood and that demonstrated common communication failures in medicine. Physician training is also different from training for the other disciplines with which we work, such as nursing and pharmacy, and our communication styles are different. Various disciplines are taught to value different styles and have different expectations of what makes good communication. Other barriers to good communication include lack of standardized tools, which will be discussed further here, as well as ego, lack of confidence, lack of experience, complexity of healthcare systems, distraction, lack of standardization, and hierarchy.[3]

There are a number of tools that can help the provider to communicate more clearly with others, to ensure that one's own thoughts are understood, and to understand others more clearly and accurately. If providers use standardized tools with one another, both the big picture and details of a message are not missed. Foronda et al. conducted a review that overall showed that communication skills are improved by training, including the use of simulation and standardized tools.[3] Some of these tools are discussed more in detail below.

The use of the electronic medical record has improved provider communication and reduced miscommunication due to difficult-to-read handwriting by physicians and other staff. Computerized physician order entry has eliminated errors due to handwritten physician orders (e.g., medication name misinterpretation, missed details such as route or frequency) and has clarified communication greatly. Tools for written clarity, such as avoiding trailing zeros, using zeros before a decimal point, and avoiding the use of inappropriate abbreviations are now often automatically corrected in an electronic medication order. Abbreviations can, of course, still lead to confusion, especially when speaking to people without a medical or nursing background. Thus, we will be focusing on tools for improved communication outside of the traditional medical record.

Of note, we will not be discussing health literacy and specific tools to improve our communication with patients in this chapter, though certainly proper communication with patients can indeed be a patient safety issue, and some of the tools outlined below can be adapted for use with patients. We will not be discussing tools such as feedback, conflict resolution, and daily rounding, which are in fact tools for communication, but out of scope for this particular chapter. Finally, simulation (discussed in Chapter 2) is a key method by which these communication tools are taught and reinforced, but it will not be discussed in detail here.

A culture of clear communication is exactly that: a culture. Tools alone are not the foundation of a system that values patient safety above all else; they do, however, give those who care for patients a common language and serve to reinforce a culture that values teamwork, clear communication, and high-quality care above all else.

Examples of Clear Communication in the Nonhealthcare Setting

Industries outside of healthcare have embraced the need to communicate clearly in order to ensure safety, accuracy, and quality, which in turn leads to proper customer service.

Physicians see one of the best examples of clear communication in industry every day when they buy their morning coffee. Starbucks always employs a repeat-back/read-back system, in which an employee hears your order, writes it down on a cup, and reads it back to you (read-back). That employee then reads the order out loud to the barista (second employee), who calls the order back out (repeat-back).

Another classic example of a tool to increase understanding is the military or phonetic NATO alphabet. So as to avoid confusion when spelling out letters, words that do not sound similar to one another (such as "bravo," "charlie," "delta," "echo," "foxtrot" instead of "B," "C," "D," "E," "F") are used instead.[4]

Finally, pilots must repeat-back instructions received from air traffic control, as well as repeat-back other crucial information, often to one another.[5]

A fairly well-known example occurred during the now famous "Miracle on the Hudson," in which US Airways Flight 1549 landed on the Hudson River in January 2009, after it was noted that a flock of geese had flown into the engines, stalling them. Captain Chesley "Sully" Sullenberger and Co-Pilot Jeff Skiles offer a perfect example of a repeat-back and closed-loop communication:

15:27:23.2: Sullenberger: "my aircraft"
15:27:24: Skiles: "your aircraft."[6]

This extremely short, simple, and habit-based, almost unconscious repeat-back ensured that the two pilots had a shared mental model. In those four words, ownership of the plane and the safety of the 153 other people aboard transferred from one pilot to another in the span of 0.8 seconds.

Clear Communication in Medicine

Some healthcare systems have taught from the concepts of "Crew Resource Management" (CRM). Based on training developed for aviation by psychologists John Lauber and Robert Helmreich, among others, CRM focuses on group dynamics, leadership, interpersonal communication, and decision-making, and allows crews to "identify existing and potential threats and to develop, communicate and implement plans and actions to avoid or mitigate perceived threats."[7] Vanderbilt Medical Center teaches a version of CRM to its staff, focusing on the mantra, "see it, say it, fix it," and focusing on tools such as briefs, debriefs, huddles, and assertive statements to facilitate communication.

TeamSTEPPS, a system developed by the Agency for Healthcare Research and Quality and the Department of Defense, in order to promote and improve teamwork and collaboration in healthcare, has been shown to improve outcomes and is based on the CRM principles. TeamSTEPPS focuses on four-core "teachable-learnable skills," one of which is communication. They define communication as "the exchange of information between a sender and a receiver, irrespective of the medium." Examples of communication to enhance safe outcomes include following up to ensure team members heard your message, acknowledging when a message is heard that it was indeed received, asking for clarification when uncertain about a message, and confirming that you heard the correct message.[8]

The TeamSTEPPS curriculum specifically teaches four main communication tools to aid in clear communication: "SBAR," "call-out," "check-back," and the previously discussed handoffs. In addition, though not taught specifically within their communication module, TeamSTEPPS suggests tools to increase "mutual support" that are considered by some to be communication tools and are mentioned in this chapter, including escalation (advocacy/assertion and "CUS"). More specifics are provided below regarding some of these communication tools.

Tool for Clear Communication: Call-Out

A call-out is a tool used to communicate critical information quickly. Although it seems like a very simple tool, and one we do every day, such as reading vital signs out loud to someone who is recording them or asking for help due to escalating patient care needs, it is particularly helpful when used in critical or near-critical situations in which multiple people need to hear the same information and have a shared mental model. For example, rather than code leaders speaking only with one or two members of a team at a time, having them prompt the call-outs by asking for status updates (e.g., "Airway status?" "Airway clear." "Breath sounds?" "Decreased on the right.") allows all members of the code team to be on the same page.[9] Another example of an excellent call-out that should not be taken for granted is during the transition of leadership from one person to another during a critical situation: "I'm Doctor Y, I'll be taking over the Code now." Teaching providers that this tool ought not be taken for granted is valuable and can be done via examples, modelling, coaching, and simulation.

Tool for Clear Communication: Repeat-Back/Read-Back/Check-Back

Repeat-backs and read-backs are used widely in other industries, as noted above. In healthcare, they are already often used in two particular areas: critical result notification and verbal order read-back.

Critical results are required to be called according to the 2002 National Patient Safety Goals by the Joint Commission on Accreditation of Healthcare Organizations. In 2004, the goals were amended to include an improvement to the safety of this practice, requiring a repeat-back of the critical result.[10]

Barenfanger et al. published a study in 2004 in which they used repeat-backs to minimize errors from misunderstood critical results. They implemented a system at three healthcare organizations in which telephone recipients of critical results were required to repeat-back the message heard (name, test, and result). The caller used a standard script in each call: "In order to ensure you have the right information, please repeat the name, test, and result I just gave you." An error rate of 3.5% was detected by the repeat-back (29 of 822 calls); these included incorrect patient name, incorrect test result, incorrect specimen/test repeated, and the refusal of the recipient to repeat the message. All errors were corrected by the repeat-back, and the time required to ask for the repeat-back and complete the repeat-back was only 12.8 seconds per call.[11] Interestingly, calls to physicians had the highest rate of errors (5%, or 6 of 95). "Although physicians received the fewest calls, they had the highest rate of errors. Ironically, in our experience, the technologists are most reluctant to ask physicians to repeat the message, but physicians have the greatest need for this safety net."

In a commentary on the above article, it was noted that the University of Virginia has a critical result repeat-back policy that requires that the ordering physician be notified of a critical result. They have found that they have a significant issue with refusal by physicians to repeat-back results, which highlights the crucial need for physician buy-in of these safety net tools.

Many healthcare organizations have recognized the inherent risks in physician verbal ordering and have put systems in place to make verbal orders safer. The National Coordinating Council to Prevent Medication Errors recommends that all recipients of physician verbal orders do a read-back.[12]

Outside of the above two areas, repeat-backs and read-backs can also aid in improving the quality of patient care. Boyd et al. studied read-backs in postanesthesia care unit nurses, anesthetic assistants, and anesthesiologists in a series of 88 simulations. The nurses and assistants were given clinically important information at the start of the simulation and then were given a clinical crisis scenario that necessitated calling the anesthesiologist, who knew nothing about the patients. The authors noted whether the anesthesiologist repeated back the information, verbally responded without a repeat-back, or did not respond at all each time a critical piece of information was mentioned by the nurse or assistant. They found that the people who repeated back information were 8.27 times (p < 0.001) more likely to know the information than those with no verbal response (3.16 times more likely, p = 0.03, for those who verbally responded without a repeat-back as opposed to no verbal response).[13]

Finally, check-backs, a component of "closed loop communication," are a tool used to "ensure that information conveyed by the sender is understood by the receiver as intended." The first component of the tool is the message, and the second is a repeat or read-back, which begins the check-back; the third component, confirmation that the message was heard correctly, concludes the check-back[8, 10]:

(1) Sender initiates a message
(2) Receiver accepts the message and feeds back that the message was received
(3) Sender double-checks and confirms that the message was received correctly

For example,

(1) Sender: "Give 2mg of IV lorazepam" = message
(2) Receiver: "That's 2mg of IV lorazepam" = repeat-back/check-back
(3) Sender: "That's correct" = check-back confirmation

Tools for Clear Communication: SBAR

SBAR stands for "Situation, Background, Assessment, and Recommendation." It is a tool that allows for concise transmission of a set of information, and it has been used for years to improve the formation of a "shared mental model," or a shared understanding of a situation, between the giver and receiver of information. SBAR allows for improved listening, clearer understanding, and better teamwork, as the giver of information feels heard and is able to share all the information they wish to convey, and the receiver of information receives a complete summary (Tables 14.1 and 14.2).[9, 15]

Haig et al. described their effort to make SBAR the norm at a hospital in Illinois in order to enhance the concept of a shared mental model. SBAR became the standard communication methodology not just between physicians and nurses but also from leadership to the rest of the hospital. They noted that staff seemed to adapt quickly to using the tool, though there was hesitancy around giving the recommendation to physicians. In order to address that, medical staff were taught to actively listen for the components of SBAR and solicit a recommendation if not originally offered.[15]

The SBAR tool was used as an "anchor tool" for team-based communication in an interprofessional leadership program. The authors studied clinician and administrator perceptions of SBAR as an interprofessional communication tool in both clinical and nonclinical situations. Twenty-two clinicians of multiple disciplines (physicians, nurses, and allied health professionals) and 10 administrators attended a five-day leadership course, including a three-hour SBAR training workshop, followed by workplace application of the tool. Scenarios were inspired by real-life situations and were both clinical and nonclinical. Both clinical and nonclinical participants endorsed that SBAR was easy to use, applicable, and effective. In particular, four main themes were identified as to why SBAR worked well across disciplines as well as in both clinical and nonclinical settings: (1) it provided a common language across disciplines, (2) it was efficiently organized, (3) it facilitated collaborative team-based communication, and (4) it allowed for use in various formats, including face-to-face and email.[16]

Another author taught final-year medical students a modified SBAR tool and compared their results in a patient care simulation to those of a control group not taught the tool. All groups were scored on communication content and clarity of delivery of information. Those in the intervention group scored significantly higher in both areas as compared to the control group ($p < 0.001$ for each).[17]

Table 14.1 Situation, background, assessment, and recommendation

Situation	One sentence clear description of the problem
Background	Clear and relevant details that relate to the situation and support the assessment (e.g., patient diagnosis, current exam findings).
Assessment	Your analysis and professional conclusion
Recommendation (or request)	The action that is needed from the person you are contacting; your suggestion for how to solve the problem at hand

Table 14.2 SBAR example

Without SBAR (nursing student)	"Um, do you know this patient? Her urine is a little dark…"
In SBAR format (nursing preceptor)	"I have a concern about patient X in room Y, POD 2 from Z surgery (S). She's not voided much this shift, only 100ml of dark urine, and she's not drinking much (B). She lost her IV earlier today and I'm concerned she's getting dehydrated (A). Would you please come assess her and let me know whether you think her IV needs to be replaced and, if so, what IV fluids she may need? (R)."

Beckett and Kipnis introduced SBAR, along with other team-building and collaboration strategies in an hour-long module, to both nurse and physician groups at a community hospital. Though physicians did not participate in their pre-intervention and postintervention surveys, they found statistically significant increases in many areas of the "Teamwork and Safety Climate Survey" completed by nursing in areas such as "nursing input is well received in this clinical area" and "I am satisfied with the quality of collaboration that I experience with staff physicians in this clinical area."[18]

Finally, one study examined a comprehensive team communication toolkit including SBAR at Denver Health Medical Center, focusing on the Medical Intensive Care Unit and Acute Care Unit. The results demonstrated statistically significant improvements in time needed for resolution of an issue and nurse satisfaction.[15]

The Institute for Healthcare Improvement offers a number of SBAR tools such as the communication tool itself, scenarios, lesson plans, and tips.

Tool for Clear Communication: Briefs, Huddles, and Debriefs

TeamSTEPPS teaches that effective team leaders "identify and articulate clear goals (i.e. the plan)," "facilitate information sharing," and "monitor and modify the plan; communicate changes," among other things. Briefs, huddles, and debriefs are some of the tools that allow for those things to happen effectively (Table 14.3).

The Denver Health Medical Center toolkit noted above not only included SBAR, as above, but also daily goals via rounds, as well as team huddles each shift and a standardized escalation tool; they found significant improvements postimplementation in time needed to communicate and to resolve an issue, as well as nurse satisfaction with resolution of

Table 14.3 TeamSTEPPS Brief, Huddle, Debrief[8]

Tool	Goals	Example
Brief	Start off a plan, assign roles/responsibilities, establish expectations, anticipate contingencies	Early a.m. brief in OR prior to day's cases
Huddle	Monitor and modify a plan – reinforce and assess need for adjustment	Huddle to review insulin management during PACU stay following long OR course
Debrief	Review team performance in order to reinforce positive behaviors and identify lessons learned for a future similar event	Quick review of resuscitation following intubation of a patient with a difficult airway by the hospital code team

an issue. Their huddles, which were less than 15 minutes and focused on limited agenda items, allowed teams to quickly share information with each other to allow relevant operational planning to take place.[19]

Tool for Clear Communication: Standard Escalation

Finally, though also not taught specifically as a communication tool, TeamSTEPPS teaches escalation via the tools of advocacy/assertion, the "two-challenge rule," and "CUS."

Advocacy/assertion is necessary when team members do not agree with a decision by a person of higher authority. The goal is to assert or suggest a corrective action respectfully by stating the concern, stating the problem, offering a solution, and reaching agreement on next steps. Note this is somewhat similar to SBAR above. In order to do this, one might use the TeamSTEPPS assertive statements, or "CUS words":

"I am Concerned" → "I am Uncomfortable" → "This is a Safety issue."

Similarly, in their CRM teachings, Vanderbilt University Medical Center teaches the use of such assertive statements, meant to "address a critical deviation from the shared mental model in a timely manner, while avoiding defensiveness from any team member" in the following format:

(1) Get someone's attention by saying their name
(2) Express personal concern, for example, "I am concerned"
(3) Objectively state the problem (e.g., concerning vital signs)
(4) Recommend a solution, ideally done using a "we statement."[20]

Finally, the "two-challenge" rule, used when an assertive statement is not successful, is meant to "stop the line" when a critical safety breach is at hand. TeamSTEPPS teaches that it is the responsibility of the provider to voice a concern at least two times to ensure it is heard, and if there is no agreed upon resolution, to use his or her chain of command to escalate their concern.

Conclusion

Communication tools are necessary to improve our skills in providing the safest patient care possible. Various disciplines within healthcare are not taught these tools during training or are taught to value different aspects of communication. The above skills can be incorporated into curricula for medical students, physician trainees, and continuing medical education for practicing physicians. In addition to teaching the above skills, though, the strongest healthcare systems should also include teamwork training, low- and high-fidelity simulation, and other interventions that reinforce the values of teamwork and camaraderie.[3] Use of the simple tools discussed here alone can help to influence a culture of reliability and safety, as they are one step toward the goal of high-quality patient care provided by seamless teams. The use of proper communication tools is an integral piece of a healthcare system's culture: They need to lay upon a strong foundation of safety that is made up of pieces other than simply good communication, but they also may also serve to reinforce and strengthen the foundation of individual and institutional safety and reliability.

References

1. Joint Commission's Annual Report on Quality and Safety 2007. www .jointcommission.org/assets/1/6/2007_ Annual_Report.pdf

2. Vermeir P, Vandijck D, Degroote S, et al. Communication in healthcare: A narrative review of the literature and practical recommendations. *International Journal of Clinical Practice.* 2015;69(11):1257–1267. [published Online First: 2015/07/06].

3. Foronda C, MacWilliams B, and McArthur E. Interprofessional communication in healthcare: An integrative review. *Nurse Education in Practice.* 2016;19:36–40.

4. https://militarybenefits.info/military alphabet/ (Accessed 4/25/2021).

5. Pilot responsibility for compliance with air traffic control clearances and instructions, 64 Federal Register 15911–15914 (1999), part IV.

6. www.tailstrike.com/150109.htm (Accessed 4/25/2021).

7. www.apa.org/action/resources/research-in-action/crew.aspx

8. TeamSTEPPS Fundamentals Course. www.ahrq.gov/teamstepps/instructor/ fundamentals/module1/m1evidencebase .html

9. Pocket Guide, TeamSTEPPS 2.0:Team Strategies & Tools to Enhance Performance and Patient Safety. www .ahrq.gov/sites/default/files/wysiwyg/ professionals/education/curriculum-tools/teamstepps/instructor/essentials/ pocketguide.pdf

10. Joint Commission on Accreditation of Healthcare Organization. 2004 National Patient Safety Goals. www .jcaho.com/accredited+organizations/ laboratory+services/standards/revisions/ npsg_lab.htm

11. Barenfanger J, Sautter RL, Lang DL, et al. Improving patient safety by repeating (read-back) telephone reports of critical information. *American Journal of Clinical Pathology.* June 2004;121(6):801–803.

12. National Coordinating Council for Medication Error Reporting and Prevention: Recommendations to Reduce Medication Errors Associated with Verbal Medication Orders and Prescriptions: adopted February 20, 2001. www .nccmerp.org/recommendations-reduce-medication-errors-associated-verbal-medication-orders-and-prescriptions.

13. Boyd M, Cumin D, Lombard B, et al. Read-back improves information transfer in simulated clinical crises. *BMJ Quality & Safety.* December 2014;23(12):989–993.

14. Institute for Healthcare Improvement, Cambridge, MA, USA. SBAR Tool: Situation-Background-Assessment-Recommendation www.ihi.org/resources/ Pages/Tools/SBARToolkit.aspx (Accessed 7/24/22).

15. Haig KM, Sutton S, and Whittington J. SBAR: A shared mental model for improving communication between clinicians. *Joint Commission Journal on Quality & Patient Safety.* 2006;32(3): 167–175.

16. Lee SY, Dong L, Lim YH, et al. SBAR: Towards a common interprofessional team-based communication tool. *Medical Education.* 2016;50:1167–1168.

17. Marshall S, Harrison J, and Flanagan B. The teaching of a structured tool improves the clarity and content of interprofessional clinical communication. *BMJ Quality & Safety.* 2009;18:137–140.

18. Beckett CD and Kipnis G. Collaborative communication: Integrating SBAR to improve quality/patient safety outcomes. *Journal for Healthcare Quality.* September–October 2009; 31(5):19–28.

19. Dingley C, Daugherty K, Derieg MK, et al. Improving patient safety through provider communication strategy enhancements. *Advances in Patient Safety: New Directions and Alternative Approaches* (Vol. 3: Performance and Tools). Henriksen K, Battles JB, Keyes MA, et al., eds., Rockville, MD, Agency for Healthcare Research and Quality (US), August 2008. Available from: www.ncbi.nlm.nih.gov/books/NBK43663/

20. Crew Resource Management. Vanderbilt University Medical Center. ww2.mc.vanderbilt.edu/crew_training/17183

Winning Hearts and Minds: Leading Change

Lynn D. Martin, Daniel K. W. Low, and Sally E. Rampersad

Introduction

As described by Deming, the father of modern continuous quality improvement, the ability to survive is dependent on the ability to change successfully in response to internal and external stimuli. The rate of change in medicine continues to accelerate at an ever-increasing pace. In order to remain competitive, to keep up with the latest technologies and treatments, and to meet the expectations of our patients and families, those working in healthcare have to embrace change, as only through change can we meet these challenges. Physicians, the providers of medicine, have historically been noted for their limited and slow pace of change, even in the face of compelling evidence suggesting that change is necessary. Healthcare leaders will need to effectively facilitate and manage change if they are going to be successful in their roles and professions.

In order to introduce change successfully and to have it become ingrained and sustained, it is necessary to understand how the process of change occurs for both organizations and individuals and how easily it can become disrupted. With some actual case studies in anesthesiology, the authors hope to share their wisdom on how to capture the "hearts and minds" for successful change in a modern practice.

Organizational Change Management Models

The earliest organizational change model was first developed by Kurt Lewin,[1] commonly referred to as the three-step model. This model is broken down into three simple steps: unfreeze, change, and refreeze transitioning from one equilibrium point to another (Figure 15.1). It offers a generic receipt for understanding organizational change and development.

Unfreezing refers to altering the existing stable equilibrium (i.e., the current state) by changing present behaviors and attitudes.[2] A primary requirement for this transition is for the organization or group to go through a period of self-reflection and involvement intended to create motivation and readiness among members to give up deep-rooted patterns and routines. It is wise to invest time in developing change programs to organize and discuss the need for change in order to minimize reluctance. Members need information and evidence showing that change is not only possible but also desirable. With this "burning platform," change can then be attempted. Finally, the refreezing stage is when all transformations are made permanent and the new equilibrium is established. This involves setting up a process that ensures the new behaviors will be relatively secure against reversion to prior operational modes. Lewin's model clearly articulates that driving forces encourage change while restraining forces oppose change. Therefore, change will

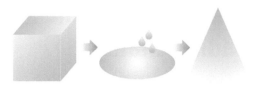

Figure 15.1 Lewin's freeze/unfreeze Model
Reproduced with permission from Mind Tools
(A black and white version of this figure will appear in some formats. For the color version, refer to the plate section.)

Table 15.1 Thurley's five strategies for change[4]

Directive	The obligation for change is a crisis or failure of other methods. This is an exercise in managerial power to allow change to occur quickly regardless of the feelings of others involved.
Bargained	Power is shared between management and workers. Change involves negotiation, compromise, and agreement before execution. Those affected by the plan have a right to convey their opinions.
Hearts and minds	Change occurs through altered attitudes, values, and beliefs of the whole workforce. This approach seeks commitment and a shared vision, but does not require participation. This positive commitment generally takes longer to employ.
Analytical	A theoretical approach in which successive advances occur through analysis of the situation, setting of objectives, establishing a roadmap for the change process, and evaluating the results.
Action-based	Change occurs by involving all those affected in a "ready, aim, and fire" step-like process.

occur when the combined strength of one force is greater than the combined strength of the opposing set of forces.[3]

Keith Thurley introduced a change model describing five major strategies to manage change.[4] These five change strategies are described above in Table 15.1.

Perhaps the most widely read and practiced model of organizational change is John Kotter's eight-step change model, described in his bestselling 1996 book, "Leading Change."[5] His eight stages necessary for change include: (1) establishing a sense of urgency, (2) creating a guiding coalition, (3) developing a vision and strategy, (4) communicating the change vision, (5) empowering broad-based action, (6) generating short-term wins, (7) consolidating gains and producing more change, and (8) anchoring new approaches in the culture. Kotter makes it clear that each step is essential to long-term success and that omitting or glossing over any step will likely overturn the change effort.

Individual Change Management Models

To address how individuals respond to change challenges, an individual change model called the "Change Curve" was developed.[6] Similar to Thurley's model, the change curve is based upon work that Elisabeth Kubler Ross did with grieving or bereaved people. Ms. Kubler Ross describes five stages of grieving: denial, anger, bargaining, depression, and acceptance.[7] The change curve[8] has four stages of change: (a) shock/denial, (b) anger/fear, (c) exploring, and (d) acceptance.

If the leader of change is able to judge where on the change curve an individual is, he/ she will be able to move the individual and the process forward in the most effective way. Someone stuck in the denial stage may need more information, perhaps because the need for change is not yet clear. Getting stuck in the anger stage is unpleasant for all and is the "danger zone" time, when chaos could arise. This is a time to remove obstacles. Change will be most firmly resisted at this time, and people will need optimal support, acknowledgement of what they lose through this change, and an understanding of "what's in it for me." In the exploring stage, people start to try on the new ideas to see how they fit. They will need direction so that their new habits and ideas are the ones that are desired. Training may be needed during this time. In the acceptance stage, everyone starts to see the benefits of change and rebuilding their patterns of working in new ways. This is a time to celebrate but also a time to make sure that the new changes are truly anchored in the culture of the organization.

Originally presented in 1998 and revised in 2012, John Fisher's model of personal change is an excellent analysis of how individuals deal with change.[9] To help people effectively move through the transitions brought on by change, leaders need to understand people's perceptions of the past, present, and future. Therefore, the leader can help make the transitions as effective and painless as possible by providing education, information, and support. Fisher's revised process of transition includes 13 stages described in Table 15.2.

A newer and very flexible model for individual change, called Nudge theory, was popularized in the 2008 book written by Richard Thaler and Cass Sunstein.[10] Nudge theory proposes that the designing of choices should be based on how people actually think and decide (instinctively and rather irrationally) rather than how leaders and authorities traditionally and, typically incorrectly, believe people think and decide (logically and rationally). The use of nudge theory is based on indirect encouragement and enablement while avoiding direct instruction and enforcement. Several examples are below in Table 15.3.

Nudge theory seeks to minimize resistance and confrontation, which commonly occur with traditional methods of changing people or behaviors. Central to nudge theory is the idea that people can be helped to (a) think appropriately and (b) make better decisions. In nudge theory, the leader/manager is called a "choice architect" to emphasize that change is enabled by designing choices for people that encourage them to make decisions leading to positive outcomes. A key theme of nudge theory is the concept of heuristic tendencies, which means the various internal references and responses people use in assessing things, developing views, and making decisions. Thaler and Sunstein[10] originally described 13 heuristics that they equate to "nudges"; however, recent work has led to two additional heuristics. The entire list of 15 heuristics is presented below in Table 15.4.

LEAN-Based Approach to Problem Solving/Change Management

Lean-based approaches to problem-solving are typically employed by Toyota. Lean practitioners in all industries assure frontline participation that is beneficial and necessary for any change management effort. Perhaps the most widely published and used Lean problem-solving/change management tool is the A3,[11] so named based on the ledger-sized (11 × 17)

Table 15.2 Fisher's transition stages[9]

Anxiety	Events lie outside an individual's control. The principal problem here is an inability to picture the positive future.
Happiness	Simply described best as "thank goodness something is happening at last." In this stage, it is critical to keep expectations realistic.
Fear	The awareness of imminent incidental change in core behaviors produces fear and will alter self-perception and how others externally see them.
Threat	Awareness of imminent comprehensive change in core behaviors is viewed as a threat. Realization that change will fundamentally impact who we are, how we see ourselves, and what is key in our personality to us. "You are not who you thought you were."
Guilt	Dislodgement of our self from our core self-perception generates guilt. Recognition of the inappropriateness of previous actions and implications can cause this guilt.
Depression	Defined by a general lack of motivation and confusion, individuals are uncertain about what the future holds and how they can fit into this future world. The belief that our past actions, behaviors, and beliefs are not compatible with the core construct of our identity will create depression.
Gradual Acceptance	We begin to make sense of our environment and our place within the change by getting validation of our thoughts and actions. We see that we are headed in the correct direction. For the first time, an individual takes control of the change process in this stage.
Moving forward	Individuals start to exert more control and make more things happen. The sense of self returns. We feel comfortable seeing our actions in line with our convictions, beliefs, and values.
Disillusionment	Individuals realize their values, beliefs, and goals are not compatible with the organization and are unmotivated, unfocused, and dissatisfied. Separation is the best resolution for all parties.
Hostility	Individuals operate processes that previously failed to achieve successful outcomes and are no longer part of the new process. New processes are ignored at best and actively undermined at worst.
Denial	The individual has a lack of acceptance of any change and denies there will be any impact on them. This is the "head in the sand syndrome:" "if I can't see it or acknowledge it then it doesn't exist."
Anger	A common emotion when moving through transitions caused by change, especially in the earlier stages. Dependent on the amount of control people feel they have over the overall process.
Complacency	People have survived the change, rationalized the events, and incorporated them into their new system. We are coasting through the tasks oblivious to what is actually happening.

Table 15.3 Examples of nudge theory[10]

Traditional	Nudge
Instructing a small child to clean his room	Playing a "room-cleaning" game
Erecting "No Littering" warning signs	Improving availability/visibility of litter bins
Joining a gym	Using stairs at work

Table 15.4 Fifteen heuristics of nudge theory[10]

Anchoring and adjustment	Using a known fact and adjusting it to estimate or decide about something unknown.
Availability	The greater the familiarity, the greater the perceived frequency and sense of trust.
Representativeness	Similarity of objects is thought to be in relation to a perceived stereotype, used when making assumptions.
Optimism and overconfidence	Tendency to underestimate costs, timescales, and challenges, and to overestimate rewards and ease of unknown.
Loss aversion	Tendency for people to value possessions far more than if they were not yet possessed, creating a resistance to giving concession or making change. People do not like to lose possession of things, irrespective of value.
Inertia and status quo bias	Tendency for people to stay committed to current situations for fear of changing to the unknown. Also caused by laziness, aversion to complexity, unnatural learning style demands, or reading the small print.
Framing	Presentation of information that alters its perceived nature, including positive or negative accentuation, association, or ways to distort attractiveness.
Temptation	Inability to delay gratification. People are naturally biased toward short-term reward and against perceived low or long-term reward. "What's in it for me?"
Mindlessness	Tendency to form views and decisions without concentrating on or even negligently ignoring real issues.
Self-control strategies	Tactics used by people to counter their own heuristic weaknesses, which then become heuristics.
Conforming and follow the herd	The need for affirmation, avoiding risk or embarrassment, following the crowd, and fear of isolation.
Spotlight effect	People tend to overestimate the visibility/significance of their own decisions and actions, producing unhelpful pressures on thinking which influence decision-making.
Priming	Manner in which people are hardened/softened or "primed" before a situation/option is introduced; it enables visualization of a viewpoint or feeling.
Language and signage design*	Overlapping several individual heuristics, design refers to the degree to which something is designed to help us understand and make the best response.
Feedback*	A critical element in nudge theory. People are open to influence from feedback or reflection while thinking and deciding, or having decided prior to decisions.

*Not originally proposed by Thaler and Sunstein

sheet of paper used by Toyota (this is described in detail in Chapter 5). The left side of the document is completed to get a thorough understanding of the problem (the Plan portion of a PDCA cycle) and the right side represents the Do, Check, and Act portions (Figure 15.2).

Problem and Current State: Start by simply stating the problem that is to be improved or solved. Clarity is critical and is achieved by going to the workplace to complete a three Actuals observation (watch the Actual People doing the Actual Work in the Actual Place

Problem Solving A3 (Plan, Do, Check, Act)				
Title:				
	Dept:		Date:	
Author:	Sponsor:		Version:	Version date:
Problem Description /Current Condition:	Countermeasures	Rationale	Expected effects	
Desired Condition (Ideal and Target State)	Action Plan			
Problem Analysis	Follow-up Plan			

Figure 15.2 Problem-solving A3 (SCH did not require permission for use)

where it is normally done). Mapping the process is the next step and involves defining the start point and the upstream customer, the stop point with its downstream customer and their needs, and the sequence of steps and the time required to complete each step. This observation will commonly reveal variations and likely many of the eight types of wastes (transport, inventory, motion, waiting, overproduction, overprocessing, defects requiring rework, and underutilized people and their skills). This is also the appropriate time to gather evidence from outside sources. Within healthcare this typically means a literature review to recognize existing best practice.

Desired State and Target: Once the current state is thoroughly understood, time is invested in thinking about the end state desired, frequently referred to as the ideal state. Care must be taken to clearly define the ideal state, including the performance targets necessary to assure this desired state has been achieved. Commonly, there is such a large gap between current and ideal state performance that it becomes necessary, if not desirable, to define more practical intermediate states called target conditions. Through a series of improvements, the team would expect to reach the target conditions before finally achieving the ideal state. All targets should be SMART, meaning the target is specific (simple, sensible, significant), measurable (meaningful and motivating), achievable (agreed upon and attainable), relevant (reasonable, realistic, and resourced), and timed (have a stated deadline).

Problem Analysis: In this phase, the team concentrates their energy on finding the root cause(s) of the problem within the current state that led to the performance gap. The most widely described Lean tool used for this purpose is the "5 whys" (described in further detail in Chapter 5). This is an iterative technique used to explore the cause-effect relationship underlying a particular problem. This method is used to get past symptoms and understand the true root cause of a problem.

Countermeasures: The actions taken to reduce or eliminate the root cause of problem(s) that prevent teams from hitting their goal (target or ideal) are called countermeasures. A common misperception is that Lean tools lead to *a* solution to *the* root cause of a problem. In the complex healthcare service industry, reality tells us that rarely is there a single root cause and single solution. Countermeasure is the preferred term as it implies that problems are never truly solved *permanently*; rather, they are attacked and improved to a satisfactory level of performance. When future circumstances change, as they always do, new countermeasures will be needed to further improve performance to the new ideal state. When brainstorming ideas of potential countermeasures, it is mandatory to engage the frontline staff doing the work for their ideas. All ideas should be gathered and, through consensus, the list of ideas is pared down and prioritized for testing by the entire work group.

Throughout all of these steps described above, it is critical to practice both "active listening"[12] and "humble inquiry"[13] to get a factual understanding of the current state and all of its problems. Active listening to the front line staff's description of the current state and its problems will demonstrate your respect for the skills of those doing the work and will allow them to share all that is good and bad about the process without fear. Humble inquiry is the process of drawing someone out by asking questions to which you do not already know the answer, thus building a trusting relationship based on curiosity and interest in the other person. For example, closing every conversation with a short summary will assure shared understanding and accurate follow-through when interventions are tested and implemented.

Action Plan and Confirmation: Once the list of countermeasures to be tried is finalized, the team will need to develop their plans for testing each countermeasure in sequence. The team will need to design hypothesis-based experiments such that success and failure are clear and ideally reached quickly. Adherence to the parameters of the experiment is critical to definitively answer the hypothesis used for the experiment; so monitoring for compliance will be necessary. The team must spend time checking that hypotheses are confirmed or rejected and, most importantly, try to understand why the actual results were achieved. Through these efforts, a better understanding of how the process works in the real world is achieved, hopefully leading to a better designed experiment in the next round of the PDCA cycle.

Follow-Up Plan: Once positive results are seen, it becomes necessary to develop an implementation plan that includes creating or updating the standard work for the process being improved. Standard work not only describes the sequence of steps and time required to complete the task but also must be documented and owned by someone who is responsible for the performance of this process or task by staff. The owner creates the documentation, including simple visual job aids, to make it easier for staff to follow the desired standard. In addition, a training plan for the staff is necessary, typically with real-time coaching of the new behaviors and skills, until the desired compliance and performance are seen. Compliance and performance are sustained through daily confirmation audits with real-time coaching as needed. These audits also represent an opportunity to identify unexpected problems with the new standard, which then can be addressed in the next PDCA cycle of improvement. This sequence of iterative testing and improving countermeasures will lead to improved performance in the process until target condition and ultimately ideal state are achieved.

In spite of the significant efforts by many scholars, rarely is change management even considered, let alone used, when attempting to change physician behaviors and healthcare practices.

Case Studies of Change Management in Anesthesia Practice

Let's use several examples of quality improvement projects in a pediatric anesthesia practice to illustrate many of the change management methods in action.

Bloodstream infection prevention in the operating room

The infection prevention team came to the anesthesiology leadership to ask for help with the problem of catheter-associated bloodstream infections.[14] Following initial hospital-wide work on the central line insertion and maintenance bundles, they noted that the infection rate had fallen by 50% but then plateaued over the next 24 months despite further efforts to reduce infections. When looking in detail at the patients who were still getting infections, it was noted that there were an excessive number of infections in patients receiving care in the OR, cardiac catheterization lab, or interventional radiology for a procedure under anesthesia in the preceding 7 days. The hypothesis was that perhaps the anesthesia provider's practice could be impacting the infection rate. The Chief Medical Officer (CMO) requested a review and improvement of anesthesia infection prevention practices.

Following a Lean approach, the first step in the process was the anesthesiology chief "going to GEMBA" to observe his colleagues' practices. This observation, done through the lens of an infection prevention specialist, clearly showed that there were significant concerns regarding possible contamination within routine anesthesia workflow. Furthermore, it appeared that the root cause behavior (gloves worn by the provider for their protection) was a potential vector for contamination. This behavior is commonly taught on day one of anesthesiology training in every program, thus suggesting that this behavior is well ingrained in daily practice and would be very difficult to change.

Next the anesthesiology chief completed a literature review to validate concerns and assist with making a case for change. The results of the observations, the literature review, and the request from the infection prevention staff and CMO were then presented to the entire department. The chief requested volunteers willing to participate on the improvement team which would develop ideas to enhance infection prevention practices without adding any complexity or additional time to current work practices. Many of the anesthesia providers were firmly on the denial part of the change curve. The first 3 steps of Kotter's model for change were critical in this process.

(1) Establishing a sense of urgency (e.g., through observations and literature review)
(2) Creating a guiding coalition (e.g., volunteer team of peers)
(3) Developing a vision and strategy (e.g., easy, compliant workflow changes)

The multidisciplinary volunteer team included anesthesia attending physicians, an anesthesia fellow and CRNA, OR nursing, an infection prevention nurse, an anesthesia technician, a surgeon, and a process improvement consultant. Confident that the team members would see the same contamination concerns, the chief instructed the team to go observe their colleagues' practices and begin data collection (baseline) on several possible process measures. Although anesthesia providers were not aware of what aspect of their care was being observed, they knew that they were being observed. In addition to in-person observations, video recordings of anesthesiologists' care in the ORs were obtained to overcome the obvious change in practice seen when individuals were being observed.[15] Anesthesia providers had the option of opting out of being filmed and were not aware of whether they were in a room with an active camera or not.

The team quickly reached consensus that there was huge potential for contamination of intravenous lines by anesthesia providers. Having the team collect this "pre-data" themselves was critical to the success of the project. A sense of urgency was created among the team members who saw how "dirty" current practices were. That team became the guiding coalition for the change.

Based on their observation of their peers, the team next began developing countermeasures to reduce contamination of intravenous lines. The decision was made to apply the new practice behaviors to all intravenous lines (peripheral and central) so that the providers would become excellent at the new behaviors by using them daily for every case and would get it right when it mattered most, in situations involving patients with central lines.

The six proposed countermeasures were first trialled in simulated cases with a team member serving as the anesthesiologist. Two ideas were quickly excluded based on anticipated difficulty with implementation for each case every day. The four remaining changes were then trialled daily with one team member in one rotating OR until all anesthesia team members and anesthesia sites had been included. Feedback from this controlled clinical trial was used to further improve the countermeasures. In the final trial, a team member serving as a coach taught one of his/her colleagues (nonteam members) the new changes in one OR daily, again rotating locations with feedback and further improvements. Thus, there were multiple opportunities for the anesthesiologists to give feedback from which modifications were made.

The final four countermeasures included (1) a new peripheral intravenous catheter start kit, (2) setup of stop-cocks for the clean administration of medications, (3) expectations set for hand hygiene after episodes of airway management, and (4) relocation of the trash bins and a new protocol for cleaning the anesthesia work space between cases. All four countermeasures were implemented as an "anesthesia BSI bundle." Instructions were given about when to have gloves on and when to have clean, ungloved hands for a clean task. The team worked hard to ensure that these new practices would be easier to follow than their older practices through site of practice job aids and readily available supplies.

Next the team presented their findings and recommendation to the entire department that aimed to both (a) get across the sense of urgency, citing the number of patients being harmed by potentially preventable infections and (b) explain the details of the new practice changes. Detailed implementation plans were communicated, which included availability of team members to coach and observe for the first three weeks, presumably until everyone became comfortable with the new behaviors. Weekly compliance data with progressively higher targets were shared with the entire department as these behaviors were adopted. The next three steps of Kotter's model for change were present in this portion of the process.

(4) Communicating the change vision (i.e., team presentation)
(5) Empowering broad-based action (i.e., colleagues in trials)
(6) Generating short-term wins (i.e., progressive targets)

Bloodstream infections are fortunately rare, so in order for everyone to see some progress, weekly process measures were reported. For example, it was reported that in an audit, 100% of providers were using the new I.V. start kits; therefore, that step in the process was a success. Finally, Kotter's last two steps had to be addressed in order to sustain these practices:

(7) Consolidating gains and producing more change
(8) Anchoring new approaches in the culture

As a fast-growing department with many trainees passing through, this has been challenging. The new "anesthesia BSI bundle" is presented to new staff and trainees in their orientation and has become an expectation for all staff to learn/use. It is one of the daily measures that are audited when leaders are making observations for their "Ongoing Professional Performance Evaluation" mandated by the Joint Commission. Through these practices, this has become "the way that we do things around here."

When infection prevention reports started arriving, the data were very encouraging. The central line infection rate in patients with a procedure under anesthesia in the previous 7 days declined from 14.1 to 9.7 infections per 1,000 trips off the intensive care unit (ICU) and hospital-wide reduction in infections from 3.5 to 2.2 infections per 1,000 central line days. This decline was temporally related to the work the team had accomplished.[15] Sharing these outcomes has also assisted with sustaining the practices in the long term.

Checklists in anesthesia

There are multiple processes involved in the typical patient's surgical journey. Each one of these processes has to be correctly executed. Failure to observe correct protocol compromises efficiency and patient safety and may lead to patient harm.

Anesthesia is an ideal lens through which to observe how checklists can support workflow, improve reliability of processes, encourage interprofessional communication, and ultimately improve patient safety. (Checklists are described in detail in Chapter 13.) Commonly, many of these processes are hidden as tacit knowledge, often within one professional group inside a team. Checklists have the ability to convert this tacit knowledge into explicit, visible knowledge that allows teams and new team members to have a shared mental model of the process. This is a foundational step toward creating a reliable and efficient system. The democratization of knowledge also serves to reduce the steep hierarchy gradients that commonly exist in today's medical teams. There's an increasing body of evidence from human factors research to suggest such hierarchies actually prevent effective team communication (e.g., speaking up when one perceives a problem).[16]

There are two broad categories of checklists: "challenge-response" and "read-do." The former requires a series of reminders to be converted into short (single-word if possible) "challenges," which serve as questions. The "response" is simply a verbal (and ideally visual) confirmation that the action has been correctly executed. This form of checklist allows teams or individuals to perform a series of actions and then stop to verify all elements have been correctly performed. Read-do checklists are more suited to tasks that require a cue before executing an individual task (e.g., PALS algorithm for resuscitation).

Seattle Children's Hospital's ambulatory surgery center clinical processes are designed to optimize surgeon and surgical suite utilization while providing high-quality, safe, and

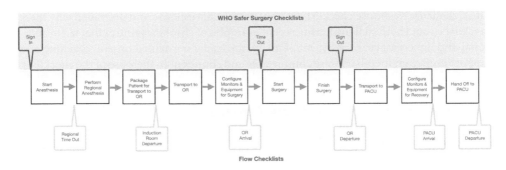

Figure 15.3 Checklist workflow (created by the author, SCH did not require permission for use)
(A black and white version of this figure will appear in some formats. For the color version, refer to the plate section.)

cost-effective surgical care. To achieve these goals while allowing parental presence during induction of anesthesia, the clinical processes included the routine movement of anesthetized patients. To enhance safety and reliability, multiple checklists were developed and are displayed in Figure 15.3.[17]

Each process is accompanied by a challenge-response checklist which serves as a cross-check to confirm the patient, monitors, and equipment are correctly configured. The checklists are reviewed regularly and updated by the team as needed to support current workflows. Up to nine checklists are used for every patient undergoing anesthesia. These are formatted to be easily read, with labels making clear who is supposed to challenge and respond, and are placed in strategic locations so they are available at the point of use. Staff members are expected to read the checklist challenges rather than rely on their memory. The responder is encouraged to use a "point and call" system when responding. Point and call forces responders to look, physically point, and verbally call out. These three actions help to prevent automated responses without a real verification step. It's a deceptively simple system, but does require team engagement to make it effective.

One of the greatest barriers to the widespread adoption of checklists throughout medicine is the culture within healthcare where a physician's individual autonomy is placed at a higher value than group cohesiveness and standard practice. To overcome this resistance, leaders and organizations need to have a "top down and bottom up" strategy that incorporates principles of change management. Leaders must be seen to be leading by example; a single leader not executing a checklist sends a strong negative message to all staff. Checklists must be living documents that are not perceived to be unchangeable. The staff members must be allowed and encouraged to edit and refine the checklists to support their work (version 5.2 is currently in use). This way the checklist will not appear an additional burden in their workload; rather, they are seen as essential checks that support the clinicians' work, prevent errors, and ultimately help create a safer patient surgical journey.

During implementation of the safety and flow checklists, leaders noted staff anxiety, resistance, and lower than desired checklist compliance. Knoster's model would suggest that members of the team did not have the skills (causing anxiety), could not see the benefits (leading to resistance), and did not follow expectations (because of insufficient action plans). Recognizing these gaps, leaders developed and delivered training on how to execute a challenge-response checklist with point and call response and described why these checklists would help staff by sharing recent examples of checklist failures that led to additional and unnecessary work by staff. Finally, the leaders provided on-site coaching and support until team members were comfortable and confident in their use of the checklists. Compliance immediately rose, self-sustaining and consistently remaining greater than 95%. Most importantly, not one single patient safety event during transport of anesthetized patients has occurred in over 7 years of operations.

Medication safety in anesthesia

Medication safety, described in Chapter 10, is another example of where change management principles are needed in order to make and to sustain iterative improvements.

Anesthesia on-time starts

This last example involves improvement of on-time anesthesia starts for all cases in an ambulatory surgery center. This became a priority quality improvement project because of the alignment for customers (patients and families) and stakeholders (anesthesiologists, surgeons, nurses, and technicians). The primary outcome measure was customer satisfaction, measured on our family experience survey. The process measure was the percentage of cases started on time, defined as within 5 minutes of the scheduled start time. To win the hearts and minds of the staff, the leaders engaged the staff in all aspects of the improvement project. First, the team needed to create a simple on-time start data collection process for all cases daily. The data was then added to the start-of-the-day huddle for all anesthesiologists, surgeons, nurses, and technicians. After the first month in which 79% of the cases started on time, the team selected a target of 85% on-time cases. Team members next learned that real-time knowledge of temporal performance was necessary to allow activation of measures to get back on time. Since every case is started with a modified WHO Safety Time-Out checklist, the team's next countermeasure involved adding a "time check" element to this checklist. Live trialling of this revised checklist led to ambiguous responses, so it was further refined to include a calling out of the scheduled incision time. With this change, everyone in the operating suite during the timeout was now aware of the time status for their room at that point in time and whether activation of their delay measures were necessary. Today, the team has already realized significant improvement in the on-time performance. By bringing temporal performance into awareness, the team is nudging its members to make the correct choices to get back on time when late. To sustain these efforts, the next steps in the process (not yet completed) are to (1) create a time status signal (green/red) easily seen by all members and (2) standardize the delay measures for each role (anesthesiology, surgery, nursing, and technicians) to further reduce variation and enhance predictability and performance. These delay measures will be created and tested by the frontline faculty and staff. Through these efforts of engaging the hearts and minds of the faculty and staff, the team hopes to achieve their ideal state of >90% on-time starts for all cases (Figure 15.4).

"Monthly on-time anesthesia starts performance at an ambulatory surgery center, since the launch of an improvement project. Note the target (85% on time) and improving trend line."

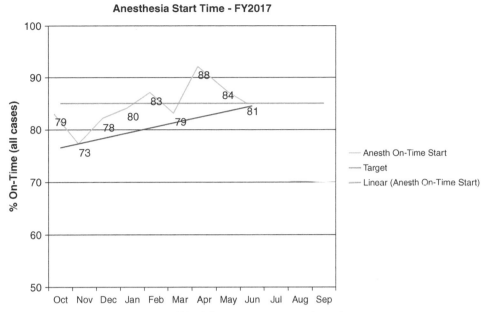

Figure 15.4 Anesthesia on-time starts (SCH did not require permission for use)
(A black and white version of this figure will appear in some formats. For the color version, refer to the plate section.)

Summary

"Change is the only constant." – *Heraclitus, Greek Philosopher*

A variety of versions of this quote from Heraclitus can be heard virtually every day in every walk of life worldwide. Like it or not, rapid change within the healthcare industry is upon us. Healthcare leaders will need to become well-versed in change management theories and practices if they are to succeed in the future. For any change to be successful, it is critical that change is not "done *to* the staff" but rather "done *by* the staff." To achieve this state, the "hearts and minds of the staff" will need to be engaged as part of an organized change management process.

References

1. Lewin K. *Field Theory in Social Science.* New York, Harper & Row, 1951.

2. Armstrong M. *A Handbook of Human Resource Management Practice.* 10th ed., London, Kogan Page Business, 2006.

3. Robbins SP. *Organizational Behavior.* Mishawaka, IN, Better World Books, 2005.

4. Thurley K. *Supervision. A Reappraisal.* London, Heinemann, 1979.

5. Kotter JP. *Leading Change.* Boston, Harvard Business School Press, 1996.

6. www.mindtools.com/pages/article/newPPM_96.htm (Accessed 05/08/2021).

7. www.stages-of-grief-recovery.com/kubler-ross-stages-of-grief.html (Accessed 05/08/2021).

8. www.educational-business-articles.com/change-curve/ (Accessed 05/08/2021).

9. Fisher JM, 1999/2012. www.r10.global/wp-content/uploads/2017/05/fisher-transition-curve-2012-1.pdf (Accessed 05/08/2021).

10. Thaler RH and Sunstein CR. *Nudge. Improving Decisions about Health, Wealth, and Happiness.* New Haven, CT, Yale University Press, 2008.

11. Sobek DK and Smalley A. *Understanding A3 Thinking: A critical Component of Toyota's PDCA Management System.* Boca Raton, FL, Productivity Press, 2008.

12. www.forbes.com/sites/womensmedia/2012/11/09/10-steps-to-effective-listening/#29f895803891 (Accessed 05/08/2021).

13. Schein EH. *Humble Inquiry: The Gentle Art of Asking Instead of Telling.* San Francisco, Berrett-Koehler, 2013.

14. Martin LD, Rampersad SE, Geiduschek JM, et al. Modification of anesthesia practice reduces catheter-associated bloodstream infections: A quality improvement initiative. *Pediatric Anesthesia.* 2013;23:588–596.

15. Rampersad SE, Martin LD, Geiduschek JM, et al. Video observation of anesthesia practice: A useful and reliable tool for quality improvement initiatives. *Pediatric Anesthesia.* 2013;23:627–633.

16. Walton MM. Hierarchies: The Berlin Wall of patient safety. *Quality and Safety in Health Care.* 2006;15:229–230.

17. Low DK, Reed MA, Geiduschek JM, et al. Striving for a zero-error patient surgical journey through adoption of aviation style challenge and response flow checklists: A quality improvement project. *Pediatric Anesthesia.* 2013;23:571–578.

Index